Reproductive Trauma

Reproductive Trauma

Psychotherapy With Infertility and Pregnancy Loss Clients

**Janet Jaffe and
Martha O. Diamond**

American Psychological Association • Washington, DC

Published by
American Psychological Association
750 First Street, NE
Washington, DC 20002
www.apa.org

To order
APA Order Department
P.O. Box 92984
Washington, DC 20090-2984
Tel: (800) 374-2721; Direct: (202) 336-5510
Fax: (202) 336-5502; TDD/TTY: (202) 336-6123
Online: www.apa.org/books/
E-mail: order@apa.org

In the U.K., Europe, Africa, and the Middle East, copies may be ordered from
American Psychological Association
3 Henrietta Street
Covent Garden, London
WC2E 8LU England

Typeset in Goudy by Circle Graphics, Inc., Columbia, MD

Printer: Edwards Brothers, Inc., Ann Arbor, MI
Cover Designer: Mercury Publishing Services, Rockville, MD

The opinions and statements published are the responsibility of the authors, and such opinions and statements do not necessarily represent the policies of the American Psychological Association.

Library of Congress Cataloging-in-Publication Data

Jaffe, Janet, Ph. D.
  Reproductive trauma : psychotherapy with infertility and pregnancy loss clients / Janet Jaffe and Martha O. Diamond. — 1st ed.
       p. ; cm.
  Includes bibliographical references and index.
  ISBN-13: 978-1-4338-0841-8 (print)
  ISBN-10: 1-4338-0841-2 (print)
  1. Infertility—Psychological aspects. 2. Childlessness—Psychological aspects. 3. Miscarriage—Psychological aspects. 4. Psychotherapy. I. Diamond, Martha Ourieff. II. American Psychological Association. III. Title.
  [DNLM: 1. Infertility—psychology. 2. Abortion, Spontaneous—psychology. 3. Fetal Death. 4. Psychotherapy—methods. WP 570 J23r 2011]

  RC889.J325 2011
  616.6'9208—dc22
                                2010004353

British Library Cataloguing-in-Publication Data

A CIP record is available from the British Library.

Printed in the United States of America
First Edition

To our boys—Henry, Ben, Jeff, and Daniel

CONTENTS

ACKNOWLEDGMENTS

Many individuals have provided help and support in seeing this book from conception to birth. We owe a particular debt of gratitude to David Diamond, director of the Reproductive Trauma Study Group at Alliant International University, for his clinical wisdom, theoretical knowledge, and passionate commitment to furthering our understanding of the reproductive experience; much of the conceptual framework we provide was derived in collaboration with him. We would also like to thank the members of the San Diego Reproductive Psychology Study Group: Carol Bateman, Karen Hall, Katie Hirst, Shira Keri, Azmaira Maker, Jean McPhee, and Leslie Tam. This group has been a wonderful venue in which to examine and expand our theoretical model of reproductive trauma as well as to exchange clinical consultation and support. Wendy Goldberg and Irv Leon also offered perceptive analyses and thoughtful suggestions throughout this undertaking. We are thankful to the following American Psychological Association editors for encouraging us to write the book: Lansing Hayes, Susan Reynolds, and Emily Leonard; their vision, advice, and patience consistently provided an impetus to complete the manuscript. We especially want to thank our families and friends. Without their constant love and support, this project would surely have faltered. Last, we give thanks to our patients. Their persistence and determination, and their willingness to share their pain, have been an honor and an inspiration; it is from them that we have learned so much.

Reproductive Trauma

INTRODUCTION

It has been over 30 years since Louise Brown, the first in vitro fertilization baby in the world, was conceived and born in England in 1978. Since that time, reproductive technology has advanced at warp speed. Although sperm banks had existed for years before this, prior to the advent of assisted reproductive technology, most couples who could not conceive naturally had no choice but to adopt or remain childless. The rapid advance in reproductive medicine has created options for family building that would have seemed like science fiction only a few decades ago, and thousands of couples worldwide have benefited from it.

Medical progress has not been limited to infertility treatment. Premature births, which used to claim the lives of so many infants, can now be routinely managed, and even infants born as early as 24 weeks can sometimes survive. The scientific understanding of miscarriages, genetic anomalies, hormonal imbalances, and menopause has done much to help patients whose reproductive health has suffered.

But along with the medical technology, a multitude of emotional, ethical, and moral dilemmas have emerged, and the psychological understanding of the impact of such technology has lagged sorely behind. Although many books have been written about how to get pregnant, or as personal journals of a reproductive difficulty, or about how to cope with stress, relatively little has been written to help mental health professionals understand and effectively treat patients in therapy who have reproductive problems.

This book is written to fill that gap. Built on the conceptual understanding and clinical experience from the Center for Reproductive Psychology in San Diego, California, the book is designed as a tool for mental health practitioners who work with patients who have experienced adverse reproductive events. Such events include, but are not limited to infertility, miscarriage, perinatal or newborn loss, and premature or other complicated births. Although these events each have their own unique features and impact, they all represent a way in which the patient's *reproductive story*—the conscious and unconscious dreams, plans, and expectations about becoming parents—has gone awry. Researchers have come to understand that these events are traumas in the truest sense of the word, involve multiple levels of loss, and must be worked through and grieved as such. Patients come to the mental health practitioner's office in a traumatized state, often suffering with symptoms of posttraumatic stress disorder, depression, anxiety, and marital difficulties.

Topics that the reader will learn about include:

- an exploration of the meaning of the reproductive story, and why it is traumatic whenever it goes awry;
- the grief associated with reproductive trauma and how to help patients work through their losses;
- how to help couples, both heterosexual and same sex, cope with differences in their own reproductive stories and personal styles;
- gender differences in dealing with reproductive issues and the therapeutic needs of both women and men;
- how to help patients make complicated decisions about family building, including assisted reproduction technology, donor technology, surrogacy, and adoption;
- moral and ethical issues raised by reproductive technology;
- parenting after a reproductive loss; and
- effects on the therapist of working with patients who have suffered reproductive trauma.

The 11 chapters of the book are structured such that the first three discuss the theoretical underpinnings of the meaning of parenthood and the reproductive story (Chapters 1 and 2), and the reasons why adverse reproductive events and the multiple layers of loss experienced by these patients are so traumatic (Chapter 3). The next five chapters focus on clinical technique with reproductive patients: assessment and treatment (Chapter 4); how to help patients grieve (Chapter 5); the impact on couples (heterosexual and same-sex), including differences between men and women (Chapter 6); how to help patients navigate the complex decision-making process of third-party reproduction and adoption (Chapter 7); and the impact on the therapist of working with this population, including the role of self-disclosure and transference-countertransference dynamics (Chapter 8). The last three chapters cover adjunctive and complementary care (Chapter 9); medical, moral, and ethical dilemmas faced by reproductive patients (Chapter 10); and the experience of pregnancy following infertility or reproductive loss (Chapter 11).

Throughout the book, the theoretical and research literature is illustrated by clinical examples, with an aim to demonstrate how therapists can best facilitate the treatment process. Case examples represent a compilation from the authors' own practices, with additional input from colleagues at the Reproductive Trauma Study Group at the San Diego campus of Alliant International University, directed by David Diamond, and the San Diego Reproductive Psychology Study Group. As such, all identifying information has been altered and fictionalized to protect patients and to illustrate the points most effectively.

This book is written with the objective of helping the mental health practitioner both understand the depth of the experiences that patients bring to therapy and learn how to help patients work through these experiences. It is our goal that through the review of the literature and many case examples, mental health and other professionals will gain both insight and clinical skill in working with this complex and growing clinical population.

I
THEORETICAL
FOUNDATIONS

1

THE REPRODUCTIVE STORY

When I entered the waiting room to meet the new referral, I was glad to see both her and her husband, as she had said on the phone that he would be unable to come. Vickie was sitting tensely in her chair, clutching a scrap of tissue. She looked exhausted and like she'd been crying. Her husband, John, leaned back with his eyes closed. On the phone, Vickie, age 34, had told me that she and John had been trying to get pregnant for 2 years. They had miscarried once, had been unable to conceive since, and had recently been referred to a reproductive endocrinologist for further testing. Knowing this, I was prepared to see a patient who was grief-stricken and in a traumatized state, who would feel as if she'd been hit by a bus. I knew that she and her partner may be in conflict, unable to comfort each other, and feeling misunderstood. I also knew that they might feel socially isolated from their friends or be unsure what to tell their parents. Most important, I knew that first it was crucial that they each have a chance to tell their story, to describe everything that happened, and that it would take a while before the rest of their history could be gathered. Right now, they were probably in shock, confused and scared; they had never dreamed they would be in this situation. As Vickie said at the end of the session, "It was never supposed to be this way." (Dr. D)

It was definitely not supposed to be this way. Patients tell us this over and over again. When asked how it *was* supposed to be, they tell us about their hopes and dreams of having a family, how they imagined life would be with children, and their assumptions that pregnancy and parenthood would happen for them as they seemingly do for everyone else—with certainty and ease. As Vickie explained, "John and I both always wanted kids. His dad died when he was 14, so he helped his mom a lot, and I am the oldest of six. I have always paved the way for my siblings, first to move out, first to graduate from college, first to get married. I always thought I'd have the first grandchild. We both love children; that's one reason I became a pediatric nurse, but I wanted to get my career established before I had my first, so that I would be comfortable taking time off. John was actually ready to start before I was . . . I never dreamed that both of my younger sisters would have babies before we did; I somehow figured they would wait a while too before they started. It's almost embarrassing; I was so naive. How can this be happening?" "Yeah," John added. "I thought for sure we would have at least one child by now. Everybody at work makes comments about us having kids. They say things like, 'When are you going to get one in the oven?' without realizing how insensitive and hurtful that really is to me."

Over the years of listening to patients dealing with infertility or reproductive loss, we realized that no matter what has gone wrong on the road to parenthood, the underlying psychological anguish is similar for all—it is traumatic. When couples contend with adverse reproductive events—which may include infertility, miscarriage, premature or complicated birth, stillbirth, or giving birth to a baby with birth defects—we hear their intense pain. When it doesn't go the way they assumed it would, they often feel traumatized and grief stricken. Their fundamental beliefs about themselves, their relationships, their sense of competence, and their future, have all gone up in smoke. This is because they suffer not only a physical loss but the loss of what we call the *reproductive story* (Jaffe, Diamond, & Diamond, 2005). Psychotherapy with reproductive patients revolves largely around the patient's reproductive story, how it has gone awry, and how to rewrite the remaining chapters.

Patients' hopes and dreams about having a family, the visions of what their children will be like, as well as how they will parent them, are all a normal part of the reproductive story: the at times conscious, but largely unconscious, narrative they create about parenthood. The reproductive story can be thought of as a chapter—one that is an integral part of adult identity—in the self-narrative (McAdams, 1993; Schectman, 1996) of one's life. Whether or not one has children, whether or not one wants children, everyone has ideas about what it will be like to become a parent. Sometimes people are aware of elements of their reproductive story: One may have specific ideas about parenting, may have picked out names for children, thought ahead about how many to have, or even planned one's whole life—job choice, where to live—around the idea of having children. Sometimes the narrative may appear not as a story with words but as more of a picture book with snapshots of a future with children: One might imagine rocking an infant in one's arms, picture kids playing ball in the backyard, or spending holidays with extended family. But often the story remains unconscious, as an intangible "knowing" that one will have a family some day, only entering one's conscious awareness when a reproductive trauma has occurred. As therapists, part of our job is to help patients understand what their trauma means to them in the context of their conscious and unconscious reproductive stories. Over the course of any therapy with a reproductive patient, details of the story will emerge, sometimes in veiled forms. It is what we need to be listening for, just as we listen for associations to dreams, and what we gradually need to help the patient articulate and understand.

This chapter focuses on what the reproductive story means, for both men and women regardless of sexual orientation, its development from early childhood into the childbearing years, and the theoretical underpinnings of this model. Introducing the concept of the story to patients early on in treatment, even in a general psychoeducational context, can be a powerful therapeutic tool. As readers will see in subsequent chapters, the concept helps patients understand why they are so debilitated by this loss and allows them to put their experience in the larger context of their lives. It provides the therapist with salient material to address in treatment and helps pave the way in guiding the individual or couple through the future decisions they may need to make. Not only does it heighten patients' understanding of their current crisis and make them aware of their partner's reproductive narrative, but the idea of "rewriting" the reproductive story can help couples better cope with and manage their grief.

The details of individual reproductive stories may differ, but for most, the expectation is that the story will unfold without a hitch and have a happy ending: a healthy baby in one's arms. Because the reproductive story comprises such a fundamental piece of one's identity, when it goes awry, as is discussed in the next chapter, the loss is perceived as an enormous narcissistic blow, a trauma to the self that can affect adult development and all other areas of one's life.

Before we delve into the theory and development of the reproductive story, we present further details about the case of Vickie and John, the patients in the waiting room at the beginning of this chapter. Their experience is typical of what couples go through when they are undergoing a reproductive evaluation and treatment. We first summarize the kinds of tests, procedures, and diagnoses that patients often must endure. We then talk about the emotional ramifications of these procedures for John and Vickie.

MEDICAL EVALUATION: A TYPICAL INFERTILITY WORK-UP

The process of being evaluated for infertility can feel like boot camp. Not only is it physically grueling, it also has a way of deconstructing one's unique personality into its anatomical parts. Removing one's street clothes, for instance, and donning a hospital gown for tests or surgery may make one feel as if one's identity has been reduced to ovaries, fallopian tubes, or sperm. The medical procedures for women in an infertility work-up typically include (a) *postcoital testing* to assess whether sperm can penetrate and survive in the cervical mucous; (b) *ultrasound exams* to assess the uterine lining and ovarian follicles; (c) *blood tests* to assess hormone levels; (d) *hysterosalpingogram*, an X-ray in which dye is injected through the cervix to examine the uterus and fallopian tubes; (e) *hysteroscopy*, a procedure that entails inserting a small telescope through the cervix to allow the physician to see any uterine abnormalities; (f) *laparoscopy*, a surgical procedure requiring a small incision in the abdomen to evaluate the uterus, fallopian tubes and ovaries; and (g) *endometrial biopsy*, removal of endometrial tissue to evaluate a luteal phase defect preventing a pregnancy from being able to sustain (International Council on Infertility Information Dissemination, 1992-2008). For men, the initial work-up consists of a *semen analysis* to test for motility (i.e., how the sperm moves), morphology (i.e., the form and structure of the sperm), and sperm count (i.e., the number of sperm in the ejaculate). Although less medically invasive than the procedures women face, providing a sperm sample is nonetheless psychologically invasive for men.

After a diagnosis is determined, women may face more medical interventions that could include taking ovulation-enhancing hormones, having daily ultrasound to monitor ovulation, using injectable medication to regulate and stimulate ovulation, and/or needing surgical procedures. Women who experience a miscarriage, preterm labor, or other pregnancy-related complications could find themselves in a medical crisis they were not prepared for. The trauma they experience becomes a loss of innocence and trust in the pregnancy process, with lasting effects on their secure sense of self and future pregnancies. Men may also need surgery following their initial diagnosis. A common problem, occurring in about one in six men, that can be corrected surgically is *varicocele*; similar to a varicose vein, it is an enlargement of the veins in the scrotum, which can affect sperm production and may be present without any symptoms (Mayo Clinic, 1998–2009).

Reproductive patients may enter psychotherapy at any stage of their battle with infertility and reproductive loss: from first trying ovulation-inducing medicines, to utilizing more advanced assisted reproductive technology (ART), to choosing donor technology. Their medical diagnoses may differ: They may suffer from ovulatory disorders, tubal diseases, problems with uterine structure, or abnormalities with sperm, and in about 15% of couples no discernible reason for their infertility can be found. It is a common, though erroneous, belief that female factors are the primary cause of infertility, when in fact the problems are equally divided between the sexes (American Society for Reproductive Medicine, 2000–2007). Patients may begin psychotherapy because they have *primary infertility*, defined as the inability to become pregnant after a year of unprotected intercourse, or *secondary infertility*, which is the inability to become pregnant, or to carry a pregnancy to term, after the birth of one or more biological children (RESOLVE, 2008).

Patients may also present with no history of infertility but may have had to terminate a pregnancy because of a genetic anomaly, or they may have had a stillbirth or other perinatal loss. These events are devastating and can have long-lasting sequelae. Still others may be trying to understand and manage a negative postpartum reaction; these clients cannot understand why, at a time when they are expected to be so happy, they are racked with feelings of anxiety or depression. Regardless of what has brought them in for therapy, however, these patients all have a reproductive story that has taken a turn in a terribly unexpected, disappointing, and frightening direction.

EMOTIONAL RAMIFICATIONS OF AN INFERTILITY WORK-UP

The experience of walking into a specialist's office can fill one with emotions from either end of the spectrum. Vickie, for example, described feelings of relief as well as anxiety, as she met with the reproductive endocrinologist for the first time. "I was excited. I was finally taking some action and moving forward to figure out what was wrong," she said. "But at the same time, I felt awful because my body wasn't working as it was supposed to, and I had to admit that there actually *was* something wrong with me." Looking around the waiting room that first visit, she felt out of place, like she was having a bad dream. "It almost felt like I was in a parallel universe, watching myself go through the motions. I was not supposed to be in *this* waiting room seeing *this* kind of doctor. I should have been seeing an obstetrician at this point in my life."

Vickie's initial tests included a hysterosalpingogram, which showed that one tube was blocked and the other slightly damaged. Their doctor speculated that when she was younger, she may have had an infection that never got diagnosed and that damaged her tubes. She commented that, adding to her distress, "I've always been really attuned to my body—how could I have had an infection and not know it? And how come I got pregnant once but then never again?" John had been devastated by the miscarriage, both because he so much wanted to have a child and also because he felt so helpless in providing reassurance to Vickie. "I'm trying to be supportive," he said. "But Vickie gets so upset sometimes that I don't know how to help. I hate to admit this but there are times I just want to escape. I tell her to try to be positive, but frankly, I'm having trouble dealing with all of this too." John's semen analysis indicated poor motility, and he was shocked to discover that something was "wrong" with him as well.

Vickie's and John's reactions to their diagnoses typify what many women and men experience when their reproductive story goes off course: the disbelief that this could be happening to them, the anxiety that something else is wrong, and the distrust in their body to function as it should. Their doctor recommended an in vitro fertilization (IVF) cycle, which would bypass her damaged tubes and allow for an intracytoplasmic sperm injection (ICSI). In an ICSI procedure, the healthiest sperm is selected and injected into the egg in the IVF lab. But both Vickie and John were overwhelmed; it all seemed so unnatural to them. They truly were in a state of shock and couldn't decide what to do.

Vickie, a deeply religious woman, was feeling out of control, not just of her body but also of her life and her life's goals. She was struggling to make sense of it all, and she was questioning her spiritual beliefs as well, unsure of her church's views of ART. That which she had previously taken for granted—her religious beliefs, her life plans, her health—needed to be rethought, and her sense of self was shaken to the core. "Although none of my close friends are pregnant yet, there are two nurses at work who are due in the next 6 weeks. In the past I'd be the one to arrange the baby showers, but right now I can barely bring myself to talk to them. It's that way with my family as well, especially my sisters. I don't feel like I fit in any more. The office is all abuzz with talk of babies. These days I've taken to going for a walk during lunch, rather than eating with everybody in the cafeteria." Vickie's reaction is to isolate and avoid baby-related events, which is common among couples struggling to have children, who often describe feeling as if they are on one side of the fence and everyone else is on the other.

Vickie, who had always known she wanted to be a mom, was suffering from the loss of her reproductive story on all levels: biologically feeling betrayed by her body; psychologically unsure of herself; emotionally anxious, irritated, and angry; spiritually depleted; and feeling like a social misfit. John, an engineer who we will learn more about later, was struggling to understand his wife's distress as well as cope with his own emotions. He was very worried about Vickie but felt helpless to know what to do, and he was also very anxious about how they would be able to afford all the treatment.

Vickie and John exemplify the emotional reactions typical of infertile couples. Although there is no comparing infertility or an early miscarriage, for example, with a full-term loss of a baby, the underlying psychological issues are similar: Couples contend with loss, trauma, grief, depression, anxiety, lack of control, loss of self esteem, and negative effects on intimate relationships. They may also face health issues, financial strains, and spiritual questions. As is discussed in the next chapters, myriad losses are associated with infertility and other reproductive failures, but the common factor for all is the loss of the reproductive story—that part of the self, so ingrained as to not even be noticed, that signals the end to innocent expectations of pregnancy and parenthood.

THEORETICAL BASIS OF THE REPRODUCTIVE STORY

The reproductive story does not start when a person or their partner becomes pregnant. Its roots begin in early childhood. It grows and evolves over time, throughout adolescence, into early adulthood and the older adult years, as people become grandparents or even great-grandparents. As such, it is a developmental theory that reaches into one's unconscious dreams, is affected by cultural and social mores, and becomes an integral part of the sense of self. Over time the story gets written and "edited" and becomes one cornerstone of adult identity: the parental identity (Benedek, 1959). We discuss in later chapters the developmental tasks of adulthood and the impact on adult development when a reproductive crisis occurs. The focus here is on how the reproductive story first takes shape—both the internal and environmental influences—and the psychological theories that support this concept.

The child's first relationship with his or her parents sets the stage for future relationships. The child's sense of self emerges as he or she mirrors and incorporates early interactions with primary caregivers. This process, the idealized relationship of the parent–child dyad, is essential for the formation of the self (Kohut, 1977). As the relationship with one's parents becomes internalized, a fundamental core of the sense of self is formed. Over time, as the process of internalization unfolds, children may pick and choose those characteristics of their parents that they want to emulate and those that they want to reject. People look forward to repeating positive experiences of childhood with their own kids and fear duplicating the negative. Vickie, for example, had wanted to make sure she had a career, in part because her mother had never worked outside the home. Vickie always sensed that her mother regretted this, as she had strongly encouraged all her children to have careers. Vickie's wish to postpone parenthood until she had established herself professionally reflected, in part, her unconscious effort both to please her mother and to avoid her mother's frustration. Hence it is one's own experience of *being* parented—the good along with the bad and the identification with one's parents—that lays the psychological foundation for *becoming* a parent oneself. Children absorb as they imitate; they may "nurse" a doll or stuffed animal, tuck it in to bed, or scold it for spilling a cup of milk. Although it may be easier to identify parenting themes in the play of young girls, boys also engage in these nurturing activities. When, for example, boys wield swords to protect their castles from dragons, it may be interpreted as their way of providing and protecting as they perceive their fathers doing. But children identify with and imitate the behavior of the opposite-sex parent as well. As noted by Hadley and Stuart (2009), "strands of both maternal and paternal identification are present, operating at both conscious and unconscious levels, in every adult" (p. 44). One can observe little boys stuffing a pillow under their shirt, pretending to be pregnant, or talking about having a baby some day, just as little girls do. They may also have a "family" of trucks to tuck into bed each night. Young children's play is often an expression of what they observe, but it also conveys their ideas of what it will be like to be an adult in the future. Playing house or donning oversized shoes and clothing is a way that children convey their interest both *in* adults and in *being* adults, and in this way the child's parental identity begins to be formed. In most cases, underlying this play is the tacit belief that they, like their parents, will become parents some day.

As the child develops into an adolescent with emerging sexuality, the reproductive story expresses itself in more mature ways. Teenage girls may continue their nurturing role by babysitting. They may not only fantasize about themselves as a parent but may also think about what kind of parent an imagined partner might make. Adolescent boys may not have fatherhood in the forefront of their minds as their interest in sex heightens, but evidence of their developing parental identity emerges in more subtle ways: Boys may continue to nurture trucks as they move from toy ones to real ones, or they may become camp counselors, get jobs, and take on more adult responsibilities. The adolescent boy's sense of self evolves around his identification with his father or other male role model, not just as a man but also as a father and caregiver.

One's self-concept as a parent derives from observation and imitation, but it is also based on what one hopes to be in the future. Markus and Nurius (1986) introduced the concept of *possible selves*, defined as the idea of what an individual may become, would like to become, or may be fearful of becoming. "An individual's repertoire of possible selves can be viewed as the cognitive manifestation of enduring goals, aspirations, motives, fears, and threats" and is the "essential link between the self-concept and motivation" (Markus & Nurius, 1986, p. 954). If, for example, a child imagines him- or herself as a pro-tennis player (the self-concept), the drive to take tennis lessons will be strong (motivation). Markus and Nurius (1986) stressed the dynamic nature of possible selves: They change and evolve over time. As the child develops, dreams of an athletic career may transform, perhaps because of competition or a physical injury. New possible selves emerge as the sense of self redefines what is attainable.

In a similar vein, Levinson (1978), in his research on adult development in men, described the construct of "the Dream." The Dream is an imagined possibility of the self in the adult world. Taking shape in the "Early Adult Transition" (from approximately age 17 to 23), it is a vision of oneself in a meaningful and purposeful role in life. For men, the Dream is most often about what occupation to pursue. In fact, men who built their life around the Dream had more of a chance to feel fulfilled in their life than those who did not (Levinson, 1978). Studies with women, however, found the Dream to be more complicated in nature (Kittrell, 1998; Roberts & Newton, 1987). Kittrell (1998), in her analysis of Levinson's book, *The Seasons of a Woman's Life* (1996), found that many of the women did not form a Dream in the Early Adult Transition nor was the Dream an occupational one. These women had "vague fantasies of getting married" and either becoming a traditional home-maker or balancing work and family life (Kittrell, 1998, p. 109). This held true for women who had professional careers as well, and although work was a central component of their lives, family continued to be their first priority (Kittrell, 1998). Roberts and Newton (1987) reviewed unpublished dissertations that used Levinson's constructs in studying women's development. They, too, found that women's Dreams were often split between career and marriage/family (Roberts & Newton, 1987, p. 157) and that fulfillment and personal satisfaction had less to do with career and more to do with relationships. As we show in later chapters, these differences in men and women are relevant to psychological treatment when they experience a reproductive loss or infertility.

These notions—the possible-self-as-parent or the Dream that one might have of parenthood—provide a theoretical basis for the reproductive story. Although many ideas about the sense of self in the future can coexist at any one time, those that endure from the past will define potential possible selves and dictate one's behavior (Markus & Nurius, 1986). Parenthood is a case in point. Research has shown that parenthood plays a major role in the self-concept of both men and women. A study of undergraduate students indicated that the perception of possible-self-as-parent occurred long before pregnancy and parenthood (Bloom, Delmore-Ko, Masataka, & Carli, 1999). Young adults who were in the transition to parenthood also rated parenthood as one of the most important facets of their future possible selves (Hooker, Fiese, Jenkins, Morfei, & Schwagler, 1996). Interestingly, although it is commonly thought that becoming a mother is more central to a woman's self-concept, Hooker et al. (1996) found that men were just as likely as women to see them-selves as having a positive possible-self-as-parent. In fact, men's sense of self as father becomes more important than their sense of self as spouse during the transition to parenthood (Cowan, Cowan, Heming, Garrett, Coysh, Curtis-Boles, & Boles, 1985; Strauss & Goldberg, 1999). An adolescent patient once remarked, "I don't want to get married for a long time, at least not until after college. There's a lot of stuff I want to do—like travel—before I become a mom—maybe if my mom had waited a while before she had kids, she would've done a better job. I know for sure that I can be a better mom than the one I have." This young girl is imagining several possible selves simultaneously: that of college student, traveler, someone who is independent of her own mother, wife, and ultimately, mother. The process of actualizing these possible selves will be the focus of the rest of her growing up, and the degree to which she fulfills them may have a large effect on her sense of herself as a person.

Important to remember is that the definition of possible selves also addresses the fears—and the defenses against those fears—that a person has regarding the future (Makcus & Nurius, 1986). The unconscious fear of infertility or pregnancy loss may be substantial in the concept of possible-self-as-parent. As is addressed in Chapter 3 of this volume, when this fear comes to fruition, the resulting trauma to the self is significant.

DEVELOPMENT OF THE REPRODUCTIVE STORY

Possible selves develop from what is most important to the individual and are influenced by the person's role models, culture, the media, and time in history (Markus & Nurius, 1986). This holds true for the reproductive story: that part of the possible selves that is concerned with parenthood. As the reproductive story develops, it incorporates not just the internalized sense of self and the early relationships with one's parents but also the society in which one lives. Environmental influences have a direct and powerful impact on self-concept, behavior, and the development of the reproductive story. The following sections describe ways in which family history, family constellation and lore, cultural norms, peer group standards, the media, and medical technology all can play a role in the development of one's reproductive story.

Influence of Family History and Previous Trauma

Trauma in the family of origin, such as divorce or death of a parent or sibling, can affect ideas about the reproductive story. "If one has had a past trauma in one's life, the impact of the present traumalike event will be multiplied and will influence one's current reaction" (Watson, 2005, p. 220). In one session, John, for example, talked about his own family history. He described the tremendous sense of responsibility that he had felt when his father died; indeed, his dad had told him on numerous occasions during his illness that he counted on John to "be the man of the house . . . set a good example for your brothers and sisters." He remembered feeling both proud of this expected role but also resentful at times that his adolescence "was lost" and that he had had to become an adult too early. He also expressed worry that he had not done enough to help his mom. As John's story unfolded, his identification with his father was a central theme. As the therapist listened, she wondered to herself how this piece of his history affected his feelings about the current crisis. How did John feel if his wife criticized him for not being involved enough? Did he once again feel that he was letting his mom down, this time represented by his wife? Did he feel that he was "losing" another part of his development just as he had "lost" his adolescence? Did he feel skeptical of doctors who were unable to save his father and may also be unable to overcome their infertility? At one point, the therapist commented, "It sounds as if you took your role of provider and helper very seriously when you were a teen. It must be very frustrating to want to help your wife, but to be unable to fix the infertility." "Yeah," said John. "Before we went to this specialist, our previous doctor kept telling us that we should be able to get pregnant, but then we couldn't; it turns out there was a lot more wrong than they first thought. It's exactly what happened when my dad was sick." As Vickie listened to her husband, her eyes grew misty and she reached over to touch his knee. "No wonder you hate going to appointments with me," she said. "You never know what other bad news you might get, just like when you were a kid." Again, this illustrates how one's family history can be unconsciously woven into the reproductive story, unbeknownst to both partners.

Another example of how early trauma can get woven into the reproductive story is Sylvia, a 29-year-old gay woman, who presented for therapy with panic attacks. Although she had not suffered a reproductive loss herself, she and her partner, Martine, were just at the starting point of thinking about getting pregnant. Sylvia's anxiety was not only interfering with proceeding, it was also creating a rift between her and her partner, who was eager to begin a family and felt that Sylvia was "just stalling." Once Sylvia revealed that she was thinking about trying to conceive, the therapist could begin to think about and listen for ways her reproductive story may have been contributing to the symptoms. The therapist did not speak about this to Sylvia at first; in fact, the first several sessions of therapy focused on Sylvia's conflict with her partner, her anger that Martine was pressuring her, and her worry that her anxiety would never abate. But as she explored her sense of hopelessness, Sylvia eventually revealed, almost in passing, that her mother had become extremely ill soon after Sylvia's birth. Her mother nearly died at that time, and although she eventually recovered, the story was told numerous times as Sylvia grew up. At this point, the therapist was able to say, "Very often we get ideas about becoming parents early on in our lives—like a story that begins in childhood. Sometimes, when something happens when you are a child, it can get woven into the story without us even realizing it." She then gently asked, "Do you think that growing up hearing about your mother's illness could be having any effect on your anxiety now?" The notion of the reproductive story and the idea of a connection between it and her mother's illness were illuminating for Sylvia. Although she knew intellectually that what had happened to her mother was not "inheritable," as she explored her thoughts about her reproductive story, she realized that she had unconsciously held on to the fear that she too would become ill, and might even die, after childbirth. When Sylvia understood that her current anxiety disorder was a part of her reproductive story, she was much better able to manage her feelings, which included explaining them to her partner so that Martine could empathize with Sylvia rather than seeing her as an obstacle to their plans.

Both John and Sylvia experienced traumatic events involving loss, or potential loss, as youngsters. For John, the most salient part had to do with his role in the family as the eldest son and his feelings of helplessness at not being able to save his father or help his wife. For Sylvia, the trauma was less obvious—after all, her mother survived—but was nonetheless a crucial piece of missing information in her reproductive story. For both patients, being able to identify and articulate their early traumas allowed them to understand their current crises and help their partners view them with compassion.

Other Influences on the Development of the Reproductive Story

As mentioned previously, although family history and the early relationship with one's parents play a central role in the development of the reproductive story, there are other contributing factors, which are discussed in the following sections.

Family Constellation

The birth order in a family and the number of siblings can directly affect the ideas one has about a future family. An only child, for example, might want to have several children of her own. Another client, who came from a large family, was content to have just two children, although her partner wanted more; she felt she had suffered as a child from the lack of resources and attention and wanted to make sure not to subject her own children to that. Conversely, many people imagine that their families will be shaped the same as their family of origin. One patient, for example, remarked on the birth pattern in his family, in which his father and his father's brother each had two sons. The patient's assumption (a core part of his reproductive story and future sense of himself) was that he would have two sons as well. It is important for the therapist to listen for references to the original family constellation because the more it differs from the patient's reality, the more the patient may feel like a failure. The therapist can say, for example, "We all imagine that our families will unfold the way we expect. It must be extra disappointing when part of your plan was to create a family similar to your own. Sometimes people even wonder who they will feel connected to, if for example, you are the youngest, but then don't have a 'youngest' of your own." When the therapist articulates such feelings, it helps the patient to know that such feelings are normal, as well as to draw attention to the perhaps unconscious parts of the patient's reproductive story.

Family Lore

Family stories also help shape the reproductive story. Hearing that "the women in our family all have nice wide hips for having babies" or that "your aunt and I both got pregnant on our wedding nights" sets the stage for expectations for oneself. These bits of family lore, and family pride, get woven into the fabric of one's reproductive identity and play a part in the beliefs that people have for themselves. As happened with the man who expected two sons, it also sets a "bar" that many patients strive to emulate, adding to the crisis when a reproductive problem arises.

Cultural Influences

Societal norms assume that men and women of childbearing age will get married and create a family. Even in our "modern" Western world, where women are prevalent in the workforce and stay-at-home dads are becoming more accepted, the cultural stereotype that "men go to work and women raise the children" lingers. Indeed, childlessness is often considered aberrant behavior and frequently associated with being selfish and nonconformist (Rubin, 2002). Women may be stigmatized as being unfeminine; likewise, men may be categorized as gay or unmanly. For those who are childless not by choice, the shame and humiliation can feel overwhelming.

Ethnic and Religious Background

Although the importance of having children is apparent in all cultures, the emphasis on women's roles, family planning, and the desired gender of the child varies from group to group. Likewise, the ideas one has about using ART, egg or sperm donation, surrogacy, or adoption can vary according to cultural and religious beliefs. For example, in some cultures, adoption can take place only within the family (i.e., a baby may be "given" to the mother's infertile sister), whereas in others, producing a male heir is so important that female children may be readily put up for adoption or killed. Although ethnic and religious beliefs can greatly influence reproductive choices, it is important that therapists not make general assumptions about a couple's upbringing but explore the meaning of their individual background on their reproductive story.

Aside from society at large, one's particular peer group can have an immense influence on the reproductive story. So many patients who are struggling to have a family comment that, "Everyone I know is getting pregnant." Of course, they may be sensitized to seeing pregnant women everywhere, but their friends and siblings may actually be starting families around the same time. Furthermore, the group reproductive story greatly affects one's individual reproductive story. A study by the National Center for Health Statistics, Centers for Disease Control and Prevention (Matthews & Ventura, 1997), found that women's education level is highly correlated with the age at which they give birth. For women with college degrees, birth rates are highest in their early 30s. This contrasts with women who have the least education, who tend to give birth in their 20s. The number of children they have also correlates with education; women with higher education tend to have fewer children than high school graduates.

It is important to remember that when patients mention that someone they know is pregnant, it is often a complex and painful experience. They want to be happy for their friend or coworker, but they may feel jealous or overwhelmed with sadness; often they cannot bear to go to baby showers or to look at pictures, but then they feel like a bad friend, which becomes another blow to their self-esteem. When this comes up, it is helpful for the therapist to normalize the feelings and help patients give themselves permission to avoid overexposure to these situations: "It is one of the hardest parts of what you are going through right now, to be exposed to so many peers who are pregnant. It does not mean you are a bad friend; it means that you are in a traumatized state. It can help to be proactive by explaining to your friend why you are unable to attend, even just by saying 'It is just too hard right now.'"

Impact of Medical Technology

With the availability of birth control pills in the 1960s, women were given a greater sense of control over their reproductive lives. Able to decide when *not* to get pregnant, the unspoken message was that a woman should be able to get pregnant whenever she decided to. Countless women, as part of their story, thought they could get off the Pill (or other birth control) one month and become pregnant the next. Use of ART techniques, such as IVF, has also had a major impact on couples' reproductive stories. Procedures that may have been ineffective even 10 years ago have been vastly refined, giving infertile couples an overwhelming array of choices. The downside is that women who are faced with aging eggs may now believe that they can have a child at any age. News items of women having children into their 40s and 50s further the impression that biological age can be defied and the possible-self-as-parent can happen at any time. The technology itself gets incorporated into society's reproductive story, suggesting that women can extend their reproductive years well beyond menopause. Indeed, many younger women no longer worry about their reproductive clock; they assume that reproductive technology will be there for them, and they assume it will work.

The Media's Role

Television series such as *Leave It to Beaver*, *The Brady Bunch*, *The Cosby Show*, or *Family Ties* depict idealized pictures of family life in which problems can be solved in a 30-min time slot. Movies, too, can influence how one might envision raising children: *Mary Poppins*, for example, makes chores look fun, and the title character's ability to "fix" the family also sends the message to spend time with one's children. Likewise, classics one may have read as children— *Little House on the Prairie* or *Cheaper by the Dozen*—all contribute to a person's ideas of family life. Additionally, news about the pregnancies of movie stars and celebrities is often plastered on the covers of magazines. Seemingly ideal and perfect, they make pregnancy and birth look so easy and convey the message that anyone can do it. Although many celebrities use ART, what we, the public, see are the happy endings, not the struggles to get there.

Thinking about oneself in the future—having a dream about the possible-self-as-parent—is the basis of the reproductive story. The influences on the story's development are multidetermined: Parents serve as role models for their children; social norms, culture, and the media play a part; and the time in history in which one lives and the medical technology that is available all contribute to the unique thoughts and feelings of one's reproductive story.

THE REPRODUCTIVE STORY AS A THERAPEUTIC TOOL

The reproductive story is a theoretical model that can also be used as an effective therapeutic device. Clients readily understand the concept; introducing the idea of the reproductive story to patients, early on in treatment, is an important psychoeducational intervention. Listening for pieces of the story in initial sessions, the mental health practitioner can probe into how the reproductive story went off track and how the patient thought it should have been. The therapist can use the opportunity to educate patients on the idea of the reproductive story to validate their feelings and to acknowledge their loss and trauma. It can provide patients with a deeper understanding of their experience, allow them to accommodate new ways of thinking, and enable them to place the trauma in the broader context of their lives. The reproductive story helps clients reflect on their past, present, and future ideas about parenting—and in so doing, clarify how they want to proceed. When patients are able to both identify and convey their reproductive story, the psychological benefits are multilayered. These benefits are discussed in the following sections.

Patients Recognize What Has Been Lost

When patients have the opportunity to talk about their ideas about being a parent and their hopes, dreams, and the feelings they have regarding children, they can more fully understand—and grieve—the depth of their loss. It is often only after a reproductive trauma occurs that some patients even realize they had a story to tell. Telling their story forces patients to make conscious what may have been tucked deep inside their psyches and feelings for many, many years. And once the story has been aired, it sets the stage for grieving these intangible and difficult losses.

Communication With Their Partner Improves

So often, communication between the couple gets distorted when their story doesn't unfold as they had hoped it would. A classic example of miscommunication occurs when a woman, who stereotypically exhibits the readily identified symptoms of depression, has a partner who takes on the "coach" role. He may feel the need to stay positive and cheer her on; he may feel he needs to repress his emotions and be her support. The danger of this dynamic is that *she* may feel as if *he* doesn't care, and *he* feels completely at a loss. The reproductive story is a great way to cut through this type of interaction and open up dialogue between the couple. Not only does each person have his or her own individual story to tell, but talking about their shared ideas of parenting and the future helps to validate the couple's reactions and reunite them toward a common goal.

Patients Feel Less Isolated

Sharing one's reproductive story—with one's partner, a therapist, or others—helps reduce a patient's sense of being alone in his or her grief. Reproductive losses create social isolation; couples may feel awkward at gatherings, especially if children are present, and they may try to avoid these interactions. It is not uncommon for patients to complain that "nobody understands what we are going through." Family and friends may feel uncomfortable in the couple's presence as well. The discomfort that others feel is evident in what they say to the grieving couple: in an effort to console and reassure, people may say things like "It was for the best" or "You can try again." These well-meaning statements often hurt more than they help. Many couples avoid social situations because they do not want to expose themselves to other people's anxiety as they struggle with what to do or say. The reproductive patient may actually find him- or herself in the position of comforting others at these awkward social moments.

Because these traumas are isolative, group therapy venues can be especially effective in treating these patients. Whether the group is therapist-led or peer-led, or is an Internet support group, knowing that the individual or couple is not alone provides enormous comfort. Using the concept of the reproductive story in these group settings is a great way to "break the ice" and establish a common ground on which to build. It enables the individual or couple to air their feelings in a nonthreatening environment, one in which they will surely be understood. It is not just a matter of "misery loves company"; rather, hearing other people's stories, the decisions they made, and how they coped, offers couples a sense of community.

Grieving Is Facilitated

It takes far more psychic energy to keep negative feelings at bay than it does to let them out. No matter what theoretical construct a therapist adheres to, talking about issues really does help. Some patients also will use a journal or another creative medium to express their feelings. The importance is not *how* patients unburden themselves, but that they *do* it. We have found that the reproductive story is an excellent way to start this process. Talking about their original story and their hopes of having children allows patients to recognize the full extent of what has been lost. Sometimes couples minimize the pain they are in. "Oh, it was just a miscarriage," they may say, noting how statistically common these events are. But beneath this rational statement, patients are often grief stricken; when they can take hold of the multiple layers of loss they have experienced, they can more thoroughly grieve, which frees them up to pursue their next reproductive step.

Additionally, talking about where their story has gone awry gives patients a sense of mastery over the often-traumatic events that are part of a reproductive loss. It may seem counterintuitive to patients to talk about their trauma; the thinking, of course, is that if you don't bring it up, it goes away. But just as the wound from a splinter will fester if it is not removed, negative thoughts and feelings build if they are not let out into the open. One patient, who lost her baby at 26 weeks, woke up each night, months later, replaying the trauma of the birth. She felt like such a failure on so many levels that she wouldn't even share her feelings with her husband for fear that he wouldn't understand. She believed he thought she should "be back to normal." In therapy, she was persuaded to disclose her story in great detail and even encouraged to share the photos of her dead infant with the therapist. Talking about her story gave her permission to release all her pent-up fears about herself and the future. Each time she remembered another detail—who was in the delivery room, the sounds, the smells—she became less anxious as she gained mastery over the nightmare of the death of her baby. Finally able to approach her husband, she found him much more understanding than she had anticipated.

Rather than avoiding painful emotions, facing them actually lessens their impact. The beauty of the reproductive story, encompassing past hopes and dreams as well as the current trauma, is that it enables people to unearth the depth of their fears of what others may think, their doubts about themselves, and their anxieties about the future. It provides a construct that patients readily grasp, within which they can express their innermost qualms, grieve their losses, and find comfort.

A New Ending Can Be Written

Another therapeutic benefit of using the reproductive story with patients is the intrinsic message it holds, which is: If we have written a story once, it stands to reason that we can edit it and rewrite it if we so choose. Not only does the notion of the story enhance the grief process and reduce stress, but it can also promote a renewed feeling of hope. It allows couples to consider, if just for a moment, that there really are other possible ways to become a parent.

Likewise, thinking of a new ending provides couples with a sense of control over the process. Most couples find the lack of control to be one of the most troubling aspects of infertility and reproductive loss, especially when they feel in charge of so many other parts of their life. Couples feel as if their bodies are failing them; no longer in charge of the most intimate part of their relationship, they must relinquish control to doctors and medical technicians. In rewriting the reproductive story, however, they are able to regain a sense of control over their future and can become an active rather than passive participant in the process.

Choosing an option—whether it is trying again on their own, using ART procedures, using donor technology, deciding to adopt, or deciding to remain child-free—is clearly a soul-searching undertaking for a couple. It's not easy for couples to settle on a clear path. It's common for people to feel, one day, that adoption, for example, is the right solution for them, only to wake up the next day wanting to use an egg donor instead. Or they may come to the conclusion that they are done trying and would be more comfortable remaining a family of two, but then, in the next breath, they choose to try IVF one more time. This kind of waffling is normal; after all, this is one of the most important decisions a couple will need to make in their life together, and one that should be well thought out.

The point is that the reproductive story can help them in making these decisions. It allows them to try out different endings. In fact, encouraging patients to "try on" the way a particular option might feel to them and to their partner is helpful; using the analogy of trying on new jeans, or new shoes, concretely illustrates that it takes time to get used to a new idea and to decide whether it is the right fit. It is equally important for patients to imagine what it would feel like if they didn't make that choice. This comes up frequently when couples are on the fence about whether to remain child-free or to choose an alternative means to become a parent. It is enormously helpful for them to imagine their story 10 or 20 years from now—as a couple with or without children.

Trying on different endings to their story allows couples to see beyond the current reproductive crisis they are facing. It helps them put their experience in context, to remember that this is but a chapter in the story of their lives. Even if they are not yet able to decide on an alternative course, just knowing that other paths exist can provide reassurance and relief.

BRINGING THE REPRODUCTIVE STORY TO LIGHT

For some patients, the reproductive story will be readily accessible; as with Vickie, it will pour out with ease. Others, like Sylvia, will gain insight only over time. The more patients can remember and reflect on their childhood and adolescence, the deeper will be their understanding of their current trauma. The therapist can assist in eliciting memories connected with the reproductive story by helping the patient remember relationships and events of their childhood and adolescence that may be connected to parenting. It is important to underline that this piece of therapeutic work is both dynamic, requiring reflection and introspection, and behavioral, whereby patients may list or delineate specific experiences or memories that are meaningful to their reproductive story.

Foremost in reflecting on their thoughts and feelings about wanting to be a parent is their relationship with their own parents and extended family. In talking about perceptions of one's own mother and father, a patient may discover heretofore-unrecognized feelings about becoming a parent and further understand why the loss of the reproductive story is such an enormous blow. If, for example, a patient has had a "good childhood" with a positive internal view of the relationship with his or her parents, it is likely that he or she would want to extend that nurturing to the next generation. Children are indeed extensions of their parents, and when the reproductive story unfolds without problems, one's positive sense of self is strengthened. But when one suffers a reproductive loss, the internalized view of the self as a "good parent" undergoes an immense setback. One young woman, for example, who was raised in a warm and nurturant home, miscarried twins at 22 weeks. Her lifelong sense of herself as a good person and a good mother was shattered: "My womb was supposed to be a safe haven, but instead, my babies died."

Over the course of treatment, aspects of the reproductive story can be elicited in more behavioral terms as well. As patients gain some relief from their immediate crisis, they can begin to recall some of their most favorite things about their childhood and to consider how these have influenced their feelings about being a parent themselves. Conversely, listing the least favorite memories often brings out ideas of what they are determined to do differently with their own children. Asking patients about their favorite doll or toy will also generate a host of memories and feelings that can then be interpreted as a building block of the reproductive story. Patients can become quite passionate in thinking about their favorite stuffed animal; this positive regression and the connection to their present reproductive trauma allows patients to recognize just how deeply ingrained is their parental identity. As mentioned earlier, it can also help to focus on television shows or movies that were seen in childhood, as these can bring forth the earliest notions of the idealized family. For men, it can be especially helpful for the therapist to interpret playing "shoot 'em up" games or identifying with superheroes as the man's wish to protect and nurture.

Although all of these ideas are useful, the timing of them is critical. If a patient is in the midst of his or her grief, it will seem insensitive for the therapist to move away from that material to focus on the past. Work with reproductive patients, perhaps more than any other kind of patient, requires that the therapist "take them where they're at," and listen for clues or openings in which to use some of these techniques. One useful point at which the therapist can more directly address the specifics of a patient's reproductive story is when a couple is in conflict. As part of teaching them how to hear and understand each other in the service of finding compromises, it can be beneficial for the therapist to encourage the couple to share these stories and memories with each other. The couple can see how their individual stories concur or collide, information that is essential in the decision-making process if they are presently faced with major alterations to their stories. For example, some people know they simply want to be parents, whether biologically related or not, whereas others feel strongly that having the genetic connection with a child is of utmost importance. Sometimes, it is necessary to have some individual meetings with each person during this time, to help each one reflect privately on his or her own history, to facilitate sharing with his or her partner. Each person's viewpoint on how to proceed with medical treatment is rooted in the individual's reproductive story; for the couple to be able to navigate change and to compromise with each other, it can help them to understand why each feels strongly—one way or the other.

SUMMARY

Like all good tales, the reproductive story has a beginning, middle, and an end. It begins early in life, when we are children, learning from and imitating our own parents on how to be a parent someday. The ideas that form and develop about parenthood, from early childhood through adolescence into the childbearing years, form a deeply ingrained sense of self—in essence—our parental identity.

As mental health professionals dealing with reproductive trauma and loss, we most often meet patients in the middle chapters of their story, when it has taken an adverse turn. This is never the way patients had thought their story would go—whether they are struggling with infertility or have had a pregnancy loss or a traumatic birth of some kind. When in the middle chapters of reproductive trauma, patients often feel as if they will be stuck in the emotional mire of grief forever. It is our role as clinicians to help them identify their losses, grieve them, and move forward with their reproductive story.

The beauty of the reproductive story is that it is a theoretical model, encompassing developmental, biological, emotional, and social constructs, that is readily translated into practical, therapeutic use. Patients "get it," and once they do, they can move on to thinking of the future of their story and what it might look like. Just as they had imagined, as children, what it would be like to be a parent someday, as adults, they also can contemplate new endings to their story. With new endings come new beginnings: These days, there are more options than ever for couples, which is overwhelming in itself, but especially so after months or even years of pursuing parenthood. Using the idea of rewriting their story, therapists can help patients safely try on the options to see which ones fit best.

2

DEVELOPMENTAL TASKS
OF ADULTHOOD:
LOSSES OF OPPORTUNITY

Many theorists (Ballou, 1978; Bibring, 1959; Colarusso, 1990; Pines, 1972; Schectman, 1980) have postulated that parenthood is a distinct developmental stage of adulthood, with its own unique set of psychological challenges, which fosters growth. The reproductive story, then, is a developmental concept, often unconscious in nature, with its beginnings in early childhood. If it evolves into one's adult life without a reproductive crisis, the story often remains hidden in one's consciousness, and the tasks of adult development, so intertwined with parenthood, unfold as they should. Individuals and couples who struggle to create a family, however, may feel themselves at odds with their place on the timeline of their lives: Chronologically, they have reached adulthood with all the outward signs intact—a sexually mature body and a significant relationship, home, and/or career, but without children, they may not feel quite grown up. Although clearly no longer children themselves, when couples can't have a child they may feel in limbo, straddling both the adult world and a place of what feels like extended adolescence. For many, having a child is the definition of being an adult.

As this chapter explores, the milestones of adult development (including separation from family of origin, formation of intimate relationships, generativity, parental identity, and consolidation of the sense of self) become more difficult to fully achieve when infertility and/or pregnancy loss occurs. Although there is no guarantee that these objectives will be achieved with a successful pregnancy, for many, having a baby can and does facilitate these goals. Indeed, both men and women who experience a reproductive trauma may feel as if they are psychologically at a standstill and stagnating in their development (Leon, 1990). Many feel as if they have hit an impenetrable barrier and can't see any way around it except by having a child. Even though bearing a child is but one way to accomplish these adult tasks, when a reproductive loss or infertility occurs, it may feel as if it is the only solution. As such, the developmental tasks of adulthood may be harder to achieve, which in turn adds to the trauma.

In addition, becoming a parent provides a person with an opportunity to repair or work through conflictual experiences from one's own childhood. Parenthood, consciously or not, provides fertile ground for reexamination of one's past. Benedek (1959) suggested that parenthood is a developmental phase in which there is potential for one's own growth and mastery of the past through the relationship and growth of one's children. As a child hits particular developmental markers, it is normal for parents to reexperience, rethink, and refeel their own lives, providing an opportunity to process childhood events, but with an adult perspective.

When roadblocks to parenthood occur, however, clients may feel acutely the loss of the opportunity to "fix" the damage and emotional wounds from their early development. Reproductive trauma can have far-reaching effects: Past hurts can get reinforced, and self-defeating patterns of behavior, both intrapsychically and interpersonally, can create more anguish and sense of defeat (Leon, 1990). Therapy can help patients work through these issues, even if they never have children, lowering anxiety and mitigating the impact of this lost opportunity. The therapist's role in making the connection between the current reproductive trauma and the patient's past psychological injuries can help patients gain perspective, better manage their pain, and find other opportunities to repair themselves.

It is important for therapists to be aware of the losses of opportunity that reproductive patients may experience, because often these losses remain outside patients' consciousness. If the therapist can listen for these themes, she or he can be prepared to make these connections for the patient, who is often perplexed by the depth of despair and the strains on her or his relationship.

PREGNANCY: A NORMAL DEVELOPMENTAL TRANSITION

When people decide to have a baby, they open themselves up to a new and life-altering situation. Just as adolescence is a time of enormous psychological upheaval, unconscious regression, and growth (Blos, 1962; Diamond, 1983), pregnancy necessitates huge psychological, emotional, and physical adjustments. It is a time, especially with a first pregnancy, when the sense of self dramatically alters. Behaviorally, one may find oneself suddenly transformed: There may be changes in one's lifestyle, a modification of career goals, or a move to a family-oriented part of town. There are internal changes to the self as well: No longer is the focus on one's own needs but on the care of another totally dependent human being. "With parenthood, the focus of concern shifts inexorably from responsibility for one's self to responsibility for others" (Arnett, 2000, p. 473). Suddenly and forever more, one's life is incorporated with that of one's child, even if the pregnancy ends in a miscarriage or other reproductive loss (Pines, 1972).

With a planned pregnancy, mental shifts occur prior to conception. The reproductive story may become conscious for the first time as fantasies abound about the child-to-be, even before conception occurs. As such, one's parental identity and reproductive story begin prior to the child's birth; one becomes a *psychological parent* well before becoming a physical or biological one. Caring for the unborn child in one's mind provides the parent with a sense of omnipotence and power. This may manifest differently for men and women. Men may experience it in terms of their physical prowess, for example, as when (in Chapter 1) John's friends jocularly asked him when he would "get one in the oven." For women, fantasies about the child's perfection are a common occurrence. "Images of her unborn child's perfection therefore become a crucial source of and validation for her sense of well-being and self-worth" (Leon, 1990, p. 19). This is one reason why premature birth is so traumatic for parents: They are confronted with the reality of an imperfect, even ill, child before they are ready. The discomfort of the last trimester of pregnancy helps the parent prepare for the birth and welcome the child with all of his or her quirks and imperfections. Premature birth robs the parent of this opportunity to gradually adjust their fantasies of the perfect child to the actuality of the real child. A complete pregnancy, therefore, offers an opportunity for parents to boost their own sense of importance, their own self-esteem, by creating the perfect child (Deutsch, 1945; Leon, 1990). On the other hand, people also may feel psychologically vulnerable with worries about being a good-enough parent; indeed, when a baby is born prematurely or with health problems, the blow to self-esteem is as profound as the enhanced self-esteem may have been before the crisis. These two opposing feelings—of omnipotence and insecurity—often coexist. Clearly, this is a time of great—and normal—psychological upheaval and change.

Because the biological experience of pregnancy entails so much physical change for a woman, she cannot escape the emotional disequilibrium it engenders. She feels every hormonal shift, every wave of nausea, every twinge of pain; her connection to the baby is immediate, as her body changes and grows. Although a man cannot experience the physicality of pregnancy, his psychological experience parallels hers. For both men and women, the psychological upheaval should be considered a normal developmental "crisis" rather than psychopathology (Leon, 1990). In fact, the regressive pull of pregnancy helps individuals to let down their guard in preparation for attaching to an infant. The parents-to-be must loosen their defenses to make room for the baby, just as the woman's pelvis must loosen and expand to make room for the growing fetus. Furthermore, in opening up past, unresolved conflicts (either with one's own parents, siblings, or other unconscious desires), the developmental regression allows for the possibility of uncovering new and adaptive resolutions (Bibring, 1959).

What's important to remember is that because of the normal psychological regression that would-be parents feel, reproductive patients—prior to any loss or trauma—are already in a vulnerable state. Under the best of circumstances, parents can modulate their idealized images of their unborn child with reality when that child is born. In most cases, this is easily achieved by bringing home a healthy baby they can nurture and love (Leon, 1990). Additionally, they can overcome their insecurities by achieving mastery in knowing their child's needs and being able to take care of them. But when a reproductive loss occurs, there is no "prize" at the end, and there is no sense of mastery; instead, there is a feeling of personal failure. Likewise, with infertility, when repeated attempts to produce the perfect child are unsuccessful, the narcissistic injury that occurs can overwhelm any positive self-worth that had once existed. It can be very helpful for the therapist to articulate this, so that clients understand why they are feeling so badly about themselves or each other.

The experience of pregnancy is not only about having a child but is also important in the development of the parents-to-be. When able to achieve parenthood, couples gain an added sense of their status as adults, a feeling of greater authority, a confirmation of their sexual identity, and a fuller sense of themselves as equal to their own parents. No longer just in the position of "the child," one experiences a shift in identity when becoming a parent, with an increased realization of separation and individuation from one's own parents (Colarusso, 1990). Prospective parents also may feel gratification in fulfilling expected societal roles by producing, educating, and raising the next generation. The bond between parent and child is truly unlike any other, offering parents the opportunity to expand their emotional repertoire of nurturance and love. Finally, potential parents can feel hope and excitement; their children's accomplishments become their own, providing a rich base for a parent's personal satisfaction and fulfillment.

Given the role parenthood plays in the developmental tasks of adulthood, it is not surprising that problems along the way would be felt as a personal and profound failure. The following sections discuss several adult developmental models. Case studies illustrate how the adult developmental tasks become compromised by reproductive losses, adding to the psychological strain couples experience.

ADULT DEVELOPMENTAL MODELS

Erikson (1963), in his seminal work on adult development, described eight stages of development throughout the life span, from infancy through old age. Erikson expanded on the psychosexual model proposed by Freud (1953) by focusing not only on the person's inner needs but also on the integration of these needs with those of society. In addition, Erikson extended the idea of development, not only through adolescence but also throughout adulthood and into maturity. Each of the eight stages has been identified by a particular psychosocial crisis that must be resolved to successfully move on to the next stage. The crisis of each stage refers to normal stresses and challenges of development rather than to a traumatic event. However, if a trauma occurs, such as infertility or reproductive loss, a particular stage may become delayed or remain uncompleted (Menning, 1980).

The age ranges of each stage have more to do with a person's psychological readiness than chronological age. That being said, the stages pertinent to examination here are early adulthood, which generally extends from 22 to 34 years, and middle adulthood, which stretches from 34 to 60 years. The psychosocial crises of these two adult stages are *intimacy versus isolation* (early adulthood) and *generativity versus stagnation* (middle adulthood; Erikson, 1963). As is discussed, reproductive trauma directly impacts the developmental milestones of each of these stages.

More recently, Levinson (1978, 1986) referred to the idea of the *life course*—the "character of a life in its evolution from beginning to end" (Levinson, 1986, p. 3)—noting that this has a particular underlying order. Levinson (1986) contended that although "each individual life is unique, everyone goes through the same basic sequence" (p. 4). He described the various *eras* of the life as consisting of *structure-building* alternating with *structure-changing* times, and the general biopsychosocial characteristics that define each period. Of particular interest here is the *early adulthood* era, ranging from about 17 to 45 years of age. Although Levinson (1978) defined specific ages at which the life cycle shifts and changes, his theory, like Erikson's (1963), has more to do with the underlying developmental tasks that emerge (Roberts & Newton, 1987). The tasks of this era focus primarily on pursuing a career, developing an intimate relationship, and raising a family.

Of importance in understanding reproductive crises is Levinson's (1978) premise of an *Age 30 Transition*. Typically a stressful period, the developmental task related to this time (approximately 28 to 33 years of age) is to reflect on and question one's life and previous choices. It may involve overt changes in relationships or career; it is a time to modify the things in one's life that no longer feel fulfilling (Levinson, 1978; Roberts & Newton, 1987). This is a time when many individuals establish significant relationships, and many couples either become new parents or consider parenthood for the first time. Roberts and Newton (1987) analyzed four unpublished dissertations that used Levinson's model to study women (Levinson's original work was based solely on the lives of men). They found that although the Age 30 Transition held true for both men and women, there were gender differences in how these tasks were worked on as well as their outcomes.

How do men and women differ in this transitional period? For men, the primary component of the Dream (see Chapter 1) is occupational in nature, whereas for women, even among those with professional careers, marriage and family are central to their Dream (Roberts & Newton, 1987). During the Age 30 Transition, although there are often changes in career goals and relationships, occupation continues to be the main focus for men throughout their entire adulthood. For women, however, this transition period takes a different path. One researcher found that the priorities established during a woman's 20s reversed (Stewart, 1977, as cited in Roberts & Newton, 1987). If, for example, a woman focused on her career in her 20s, marriage and motherhood may become a priority in her 30s, and vice versa. Indeed, what may have been previously satisfying for women loses its appeal (Kittrell, 1998; Levinson, 1996). Other research suggests that rather than reversing career or family, women want to add that piece that had previously been neglected (Furst, 1983, as cited in Roberts & Newton, 1987). In either scenario, if there is a pregnancy demise or an infertility problem, the task of this transition may be delayed or uncompleted. One may have difficulty moving on to the next structure-building phase of one's life if the transition to having a family is complicated and obscured. This may present in the therapeutic setting in any number of ways: depression, anxiety, relationship issues, or dissatisfaction in the work environment.

The work of Colarusso and Nemiroff (1987) is also based on dividing the life cycle into stages: early (ages 20–40 years), middle (ages 40–60 years), late (ages 60–80 years), and late–late (ages over 80 years). More important, however, are the adult developmental tasks, "major, universal themes that are engaged in thought and usually in action by every adult" (Colarusso & Nemiroff, 1987, p. 1265), which, as they noted, can overlap stages. One can become a parent, for example, as a teenager, or in the early, middle, or even late adulthood stage. Conceptually, this relates directly to the idea of reproductive story. The fact that individuals think about being a parent, whether they have children or not, whether they want children or not, speaks to the importance of the role of parental identity in adult development. For the clinician, understanding the adult tasks corresponding to a particular age range can help him or her conceptualize the needs of a particular client. Thus, if a 33-year-old woman without children presents with depression, the mental health professional should consider the importance of parenthood in her development, even if she has chosen to remain child-free.

Additionally, Colarusso (1990) viewed parenthood as a pivotal point in a person's life. Parenthood can be seen as a catalyst in redefining one's relation to one's family of origin as well as one's family of procreation. It is a time of growth and change in a person's identity and, as such, can contribute to the adult developmental task of separation and individuation. It stands to reason that if there are struggles along the way to becoming a parent, there will be consequences for the developmental tasks of adulthood.

The following sections discuss the major developmental tasks of young and middle adulthood in more detail. Keep in mind that many of the symptoms that patients present may be related to or caused by a failure to fully achieve these tasks because of reproductive trauma.

DEVELOPMENTAL TASKS OF ADULTHOOD

Formation of Intimate Relationships

Key to the development of young adults is the establishment of meaningful and close relationships with a life partner (Arnett, 2000; Colarusso & Nemiroff, 1987; Erikson, 1963; Levinson, 1978). Socially sanctioned, marriage is traditionally the means by which couples work on their intimate relationship, but certainly not the only way. Beyond physical and sexual attraction, relationships deepen as couples share experiences, reveal private fears and fantasies, and assume positive, supportive roles in each other's lives (Newman & Newman, 1987). It is the psychological attachment to another person that is the basis of intimacy. One common result of the intimate connection with a partner is the wish to create a family together. Indeed, the couple's attitude toward having and raising children can be central to the relationship. As discussed previously, each person in the dyad has his or her unique reproductive story, which can either mesh or conflict with the other. Creating a family has the potential to bond the couple in new and more meaningful ways.

An important point bears mention here. In the early phases of a love relationship, many people describe feeling euphoric, as if they are in a bubble that contains only themselves and their new love (Hendrix, 1988). As this phase progresses normally into the more sustainable form of an ongoing relationship, one that incorporates each other's flaws and imperfections, members of the couple may find themselves missing the unique sense of intimacy that new love creates. Although generally it is ill-advised for couples to have a child to fill an unhealthy void in their relationship, in healthy relationships having a child together allows both members of the couple not only to reconnect with each other but to experience anew the thrill and self-validation of feeling truly intimate with another human being, in this case, the baby. When couples are unable to experience this readily, they may become more aware of and despondent about the distance within their relationship, even it is perfectly normal.

The early years of a relationship are typically a time when couples learn to adapt to and compromise with each other. If they meet at the younger end of the age spectrum, they may have time to work out the "bugs" in the relationship before going on to have children. But because more and more people in Western cultures delay marriage and consequently childbearing,[1] they may not have time to adjust fully to their lives together before starting a family. Although the peak of a woman's fertility is in her mid- to late-20s, she may be pursuing her education or career during this time and may not be ready to be involved in a serious relationship, let alone have children. She may be waiting for "Mr. Right," who may not come along until her 40s. Or, as a consequence of the Age 30 Transition (Levinson, 1978), she may be reevaluating her current relationship. This may culminate in separating from her partner, perhaps developing a new significant relationship, and (if there were not yet children involved) further delaying childbearing. Couples who meet later in life may find themselves desperate to have children quickly and may plunge into baby-making while in the midst of fine-tuning the relationship. If the couple experiences infertility or miscarriage, the risk of which increases with age, their relationship may be put to the test, resulting in a strain on their intimacy.

A reproductive failure at this point in one's development may result in the negative consequence of Erikson's theory, namely, isolation (Menning, 1980). Indeed, a common complaint for those experiencing a reproductive trauma is the loneliness they feel. Unfortunately, close friendships may break down with misunderstandings and resentments. In an effort to protect themselves from greater hurt, couples may find themselves withdrawing from those close to them. The retreat from others may happen outside of the relationship—with friends, colleagues, and even family—but often takes place within the relationship as well. Couples often confuse what has happened to them, that is, their reproductive trauma, with the actual foundations of their relationship. Under the stress of their experience, they retreat from each other. Their relationship may be at stake not because of an inherent defect in their bond but because of the pressures the crisis has put on their intimate connection.

---

[1]Between 1991 and 2001, the number of 35- to 39-year-old women having their first child increased 36%, while first births for women ages 40 to 44 rose 70% (Heffner, 2004).

Giving to the Next Generation

Erikson (1963) described middle adulthood (ages 34–60 years) as a time when careers become more established, the intimate relationship continues to mature, and the developmental focus moves from *creating* a family to *raising* a family. Since the 1950s, however, when Erikson's developmental model was first published, lifestyle changes have taken place to make it more common for couples to attempt to have their first child in their late 30s or 40s. The delays in forming intimate relationships just discussed, the demands of higher education and career goals, the need for a two-income family, and advances in reproductive medicine and health care in general, have all contributed to the notion that childbearing can wait. Although the age range that Erikson proposed may have shifted, the psychological task of generativity remains the same: providing for the next generation versus feelings of stagnation. Generativity can take on many forms: One can give to future generations by mentoring a young coworker, researching a cure for a disease, coaching a Little League team, volunteering to tutor a child, or passing on a family recipe to a niece or nephew. Although there are innumerable, creative ways in which one can involve oneself with subsequent generations, raising a child is often seen as the most direct, comprehensive method. Making decisions for a child's life, sharing and teaching him or her about the world based on one's knowledge and personal experiences, captures the essence of generativity. It ranges from providing a child with basic knowledge (e.g., how to tie one's shoes, how to bake cookies, how to ride a bike), to modeling interpersonal skills (e.g., how to cope with hurt feelings, how to soothe oneself, how to compromise and get along with others), to providing him or her with a philosophical outlook on life (e.g., how to find meaning, compassion, and joy). The daily interaction with a child provides the forum for generativity; it may involve conscious decision making but, more often than not, it is the unconscious process of being with children that molds them and helps them develop into the adults of the future.

Clinically, the extent to which patients view having a child as the only way they feel generative will intensify the pressure they feel when conception eludes them. The therapist can help patients see the ways in which the narrow definition of generativity limits them. As we think back to John, for example, he realized that having a biological child was particularly salient because his father had died. He felt especially pressured to have a son, "to carry on the family line" as if he owed it to his father. When the therapist underlined this dynamic for John, he was able to be more open to other ways to "carry on for the future."

The flip side of generativity is stagnation (Erikson, 1963). Patients who are unable to have children complain that they feel stuck, as if their life was on hold. Unable to move forward, they feel trapped, depressed, and have difficulty seeing what the future might hold as they struggle to create a family. Their reproductive story has yet to be rewritten, and they may feel lost as to what path to take. We often see infertility patients, for example, who feel they cannot stop medical treatment, even briefly, to catch their breath and think about other options. They may be on their seventh or eighth in vitro fertilization (IVF) cycle and still want to do another, despite their doctor's advice against this. Rather than consider other solutions, they remain stuck on the treatment treadmill.

Other areas of the couple's life may also be at a standstill during this time. For instance, they may be reluctant to move ("We just can't leave our doctor and start all over"), to take a promotion ("I can't take on more responsibility which could make it more difficult to take time off work for treatment"), or even to take a vacation ("How can we plan a trip? She may be pregnant and be unable to fly"). Couples feel that they can't move forward or go back to the carefree feelings that preceded their trauma—they feel truly stagnant. The therapist's role can be vital in helping patients see the options that are open to them, not just in terms of family planning but in the other aspects of their lives as well.

The Ongoing Process of Separation and Individuation

As one develops from infancy through adulthood, the process of becoming one's own person—both self-reliant yet interdependent on others—continues. In infancy, there is a total dependency on one's parents for nurturance and care. Mahler, Pine, and Bergman (1975) described the first individuation process in early childhood; Beginning at 4 or 5 months old, children become aware of themselves as separate from the primary caregiver and develop the ability to relate to others. In adolescence, a time of enormous physical as well as psychological change, the sense of self takes clearer shape. Blos (1967) described adolescence as the second individuation process: In their quest to grow up and form their own identity, children turn away from their parents as their primary objects and look to friends, teachers, and the outside world for guidance and identification.

Colarusso (1990) proposed a third individuation phase, motivated by the experience of parenthood. Assuming the position of parent allows for a developmental shift in the sense of self from child to adult. Parenthood "is often sufficient for marking a subjective sense of adult status" (Arnett, 2000, p. 473). It's as if one gets to move from the "kids' table" to the "grown-ups' table." In one's new role as parent, one can finally be on par with one's own parents as equals: An adult who now shares the common experience of creating a family.

The third individuation phase also allows parents to reexperience their own earlier developmental trials as their offspring progress through the maturation process (Rubin, 2002). With each critical period of the child's development, from infancy through adolescence and beyond, memories of the parents' own experiences corresponding to that time in their child's life naturally emerge (Benedek, 1970). For example, the pain of watching one's child break down in tears when dropped off at day care may rekindle separation-anxiety feelings from one's own childhood. Not only can this increase empathy for the child's plight, but it also can allow the parent to understand his or her own experience from a new, adult outlook. The adult may feel the regressive pull of his or her personal childhood events but also can experience them with a sense of progression, as these memories are worked through in a new light. Parents who are able to resolve these developmental challenges can achieve a new degree of psychological integration and perspective on their past (Parens, 1975).

Sylvia, the patient who presented with panic attacks (Chapter 1), was "stuck" in her progression into parenthood due to incomplete separation from her mother. Her early identification with her sick mother had translated into a fear of becoming pregnant. Her partner experienced this as "stalling" and thwarting her own readiness to move forward into the next stage of development. It was only when Sylvia was able to recognize the ways she had not individuated from her mother that she was able to complete this process and become a mother in her own right. The question, then, is what happens to the individual or couple who is not able to achieve parenthood? Here is yet another loss of opportunity—both the possibility of parity with one's own parents and the chance for individual growth are hampered. Certainly, many individuals and couples *choose* to be child-free; does this mean that they are not able to realize these adult developmental tasks? Clearly, parenthood is but one avenue that can lead to resolution of these tasks: to feel on par with one's parents and to feel fully adult. Succeeding in one's career; being financially responsible; maintaining a home; mentoring young people; spending time with nieces, nephews, or other children; coaching; community service—these are all ways in which people can actualize themselves as adults and give to the next generation. Nevertheless, although the maturation process for adults is clearly based on many factors, having a child—and the reciprocal interaction between parent and child—is still viewed as one of the most tangible ways to achieve a sense of adulthood (Parens, 1975).

Needless to say, the difference between voluntary and involuntary childlessness is enormous. The issue at hand is about choice; the voluntarily child-free make a conscious decision about their future, whereas those who are childless because of reproductive difficulties feel their future is out of their control. However, whether or not one wants a child, or has a child, everyone has a reproductive story that shapes this decision-making process. Opting not to have children brings an aspect of the reproductive story into full awareness; it requires active consideration and comes with its own set of challenges that defy societal norms and expectations. These individuals choose to achieve the adult developmental milestones in unique and creative ways. It is when parenthood is desired but doesn't come to fruition that there is a greater risk of developmental disruption.

Choice and control are critical components of one's sense of well-being in all aspects of life, but especially when it comes to reproduction. The decision to have a baby triggers a normal psychological regression, as one must let down one's usual defenses to open the way for attachment to an infant. The individual or couple who is childless, but not by choice, can therefore be thought of as having a *crisis within a crisis* (Morse & Van Hall, 1987): They are in the throes of the normal developmental challenges of shifting into the role of parenthood while at the same time they are thrust into the trauma of reproductive failure and loss. Involuntary childlessness can cause one to feel regressed and childlike, but without yielding the forward progression that naturally occurs from reworking the past. Therapeutically this is important because when patients seek psychological help for a reproductive trauma they are already in a compromised, regressed, and vulnerable state (Rubin, 2002).

Consolidation of Adult Identity

Because the reproductive story is such a fundamental building block of the self, even when one does not want children, it stands to reason that when the story goes awry, one's self-esteem is greatly affected. With the loss of one's parental identity, so core to the sense of self, a debilitating narcissistic injury can occur. The inability to reach one's goal of parenthood as one had hoped is devastating (Bernstein, Potts, & Mattox, 1985; Mazor, 1984; Pines, 1990), partly because losing the fantasy of the ideal story is equivalent to losing a part of oneself (Mahlstedt, 1994). Reproductive trauma triggers an identity crisis that can leave patients confused and disoriented. Their sense of self must shift from healthy/normal to patient, from someone who is "trying" to someone who has "failed" to conceive, from a parent-to-be to someone grieving a child who never was. Developmentally, this is a time when the structure of one's life as an adult is being built. There are initial ventures into one's chosen occupation, and a sense of oneself as more independent from the family of origin. This may entail financial independence as well as the development of significant intimate relationship(s) outside the family of origin. With infertility and/or pregnancy demise, however, the strength and stability of one's adult identity may be greatly compromised. We have heard from numerous patients, often accomplished professionals, that during infertility or after a reproductive loss they lose confidence in themselves at work, with friends, and in their ability to make the right choice, even the simplest of decisions. In fact, one's identity may go from "healthy/normal" to "patient/failure" in a flash, and, as we discuss later in Part II, Counseling the Reproductive Patient, this can have a profound effect on returning to a sense of normalcy, that is, returning to the progression of one's adult identity.

The following case illustrates how the adult developmental tasks can be expressed in the effort to have a child. If the therapist is aware of the under-lying losses of opportunity faced by reproductive patients, she or he will be in a position to articulate and empathize with them as themes reveal themselves, and thereby to facilitate the grieving process. This allows patients to consider other ways of achieving these goals, whether by alternative family building or in other life activities.

CASE ILLUSTRATION: ISABEL AND PAUL

Isabel and Paul came for therapy after 3 years of infertility. She described feeling depressed and anxious; they were arguing a lot, which was uncharac-teristic of them. As the therapist got to know them, she came to see that this couple was struggling not only with the stress of their experience, but also with how their efforts to feel actualized as adults were being thwarted. They were confused and scared, and their usual ways of coping with stress were not working.

Intimate Relationships

One of the most important developmental tasks of adulthood is the experience of forming an intimate relationship. As Isabel described her history, she revealed that, until she met Paul, this had been a difficult step for her.

Isabel, a high school Spanish teacher, had been married once before in her early 20s. Her parents emigrated from Mexico before Isabel was born. They had three older children when they arrived, and then had Isabel and her two sisters. Isabel was raised bilingual, speaking Spanish at home and English at school. She met her first husband during her senior year in high school, decided to go to a local college so that she could be near him, and then got married at age 20. Isabel was young and very much in love with Ron and recognized, in retrospect, that they had never really discussed the "big issues" prior to marrying: children, religion, and plans for the future. Ron had presumed they would move to the East Coast, where his job prospects were better, but Isabel, who was very close to her parents, could not imagine leaving them. She also presumed that he would want kids, even though he had told her repeatedly that he "probably didn't." As the oldest of four, Ron had often been responsible for his siblings while his parents worked and felt as if he had already raised a family. From the standpoint of her youthful idealism, Isabel had assumed that Ron would change his mind.

"I really tried to make things work with Ron," Isabel explained to the therapist. "I guess I thought I could change him, but it became clear that he was as committed to his choice as I was to mine. Even though I wanted kids more than anything, the thought of putting them through the trauma of a divorce scared me." For Isabel, having a child with Ron had been part of how she defined intimacy with him; when he did not share this vision, the couple grew distant and ultimately separated. Although Isabel and her first husband did not experience infertility, the disparity in their reproductive stories created a loss of opportunity for intimacy.

Separation and Individuation

Thirty-eight when she entered therapy, Isabel felt like her life was getting away from her, that her biological clock was winding down. During the painful divorce, Isabel's relationship with her parents had become strained. Devout Catholics, they did not understand or accept either Ron's refusal to have children or their daughter's decision to divorce. Furthermore, they now had three grandchildren, with two more on the way, and were very preoccupied with them. Feeling estranged from her family, rather than involve her parents in wedding plans, Isabel and Paul eloped.

Paul's background was very different from Isabel's. Born to well-to-do, educated parents, he was an only child; he attended private schools and traveled the world with his parents. Shy as a child and most comfortable with adults, he wanted for nothing, but he remembered feeling lonely and envious of his friends who had siblings. In his reproductive story, he determined that when he grew up he would have several children and create the family he had always wanted. On this, he and Isabel were in total agreement.

The shock came when they were diagnosed with infertility. Because of her cultural and religious upbringing, Isabel was ambivalent about using reproductive technology: On the one hand, it offered an incredible opportunity, but on the other hand she worried that it would alienate her even more from her family and their beliefs. Isabel would sometimes cry for hours at a time, leaving Paul unsure of how to help. Attending her family gatherings became unbearable; given the tension between Isabel and her parents and because of the joy that her whole family expressed over the births of the various grand-children, Isabel did not feel comfortable sharing her problems with them and avoided family events as much as possible. She withdrew from them as she also withdrew from Paul, when she experienced him as unable to sooth her. From Paul's point of view, although he could understand how Isabel felt, he hated the isolation and missed the big, raucous family events that he enjoyed with Isabel's siblings. He resented her crying, was dragged down by her depression, and felt helpless to comfort his wife.

When we consider that one way to separate and individuate from one's family of origin is to form an intimate relationship, the strain between Isabel and Paul takes on added meaning. Isabel had felt proud of the way she had carefully considered all the "big issues" before she married Paul—it felt like a huge developmental step that helped confirm her sense of maturity, in contrast to the "youthful idealism" she relied on when she married Ron. When her marriage to Paul faltered, however, it triggered further self-doubt, which had a regressive effect: Maybe she wasn't as mature as she had thought . . . maybe her parents had been right that she should not have divorced Ron . . . maybe she just was incapable of having a loving relationship. Isabel had come to the marriage—and the infertility—in an already vulnerable state, feeling like a failure from her divorce and feeling pressured to begin a family as soon as possible. Infertility threw her into a tailspin, and many of the pent-up feelings of sadness, inadequacy, and anger from her first marriage and from her alien-ation from her parents came pouring out.

Simultaneously, and with painful irony, her distance from her husband and parents made Isabel long for a baby even more. What Isabel did not yet understand was that being alienated from her parents was not the same as being psychologically separate from them. She experienced their separateness as a rift, rather than as mature autonomy. Without a baby and with fractures in her important relationships, Isabel's adult development felt significantly compromised. Although she was 38, Isabel had not fully come into her own and still felt a need for approval from her family of origin; she felt hurt and angry with them, even though it was she who had defensively pulled away from them. Unconsciously, Isabel needed to become a parent herself, to feel fully adult and autonomous from her family.

Adult Identity

Isabel's divorce and infertility dealt a blow to her sense of self as well. Her cultural and religious upbringing had a powerful influence on her worldview and self-image as a "nice person who did the right thing." The loss of her first marriage, the estrangement from her family of origin, as well as problems with conception, all contributed to an enormous narcissistic injury.

Although she liked her job, and did well at it, she had never viewed herself as the "careerist" type, longing to be an at-home mother instead. After her divorce, she felt set adrift, untethered to her identity, and pushed off the orbit of her adult development.

Traumatized by the breakup, Isabel was cautious for a long time about getting involved with anyone else. After a number of years of anxious dating, while in her mid-30s she finally met Paul, a medical researcher, through mutual friends. This time, she made sure that her partner shared her dream of having children. Paul and Isabel married a year later and, because of her age, decided to start their family right away. Isabel opted to leave her corporate job for one that was less demanding, so "that I could enjoy my pregnancy. I planned not to work when I had kids anyway, so it made sense to scale down." This was a relief to her because she had never felt a strong sense of identity in her professional role, which she had had to rely on after her divorce.

Paul, on the other hand, searched hard for a better job in which he could earn more money in preparation for being the sole breadwinner. They also sold their downtown condo and bought a home in a suburb that was known for its excellent schools. "We were ready," said Paul. "We were both so excited." Through these choices, Isabel and Paul were gradually moving into a new sense of adulthood, with a more focused sense of who they were. They were both preparing for their idealized view of parenthood, Paul by solidifying his image of himself as the provider for his family, and Isabel by embracing more fully her self-image as an involved, emotionally available mother.

Three years later, pregnancy continued to elude them. Isabel was in disbelief: "How can this be happening? I have given up so much, and have nothing to show for it. And every day, I have to pass the preschool on my way home—if I had gotten pregnant as planned, my baby would've been old enough to go there already!" During this time, two of Isabel's sisters had babies, and Paul's best friend was on his third child. "I know our parents are concerned about us," said Isabel, "but the fact is, they are completely focused on their grandchildren. I feel like I am being left in the dust."

Paul and Isabel feel as if their developmental train has been derailed. They cannot yet see that, although their reproductive story is diverging from its expected track, they are taking a detour but have not in fact crashed. Their story's resolution has not yet been written, and they cannot foresee how they will complete their growing up.

Generativity

Paul felt enormous pressure, both from within himself and from his parents, to have a biological child. As an only child, it was important to him to have at least one heir, so that his family lineage would not come to an end. He had worked hard as an adult to become a successful professional, and to maintain his parent's approval, but, without being able to provide them with a grandchild, he felt that none of his accomplishments mattered. He, too, felt isolated and longed for the closeness with a child; he also felt a strong wish and need to leave something of himself for the future. It was not only his name that Paul wished to carry on: He felt that he had a great deal to offer a child, things he wanted to teach, interests and values he wanted to share. This is exactly what Erikson (1963) meant when he talked about generativity.

THE THERAPIST'S EXPERIENCE

As she listened to Isabel and Paul, the therapist was acutely aware of how complex and multidetermined their reproductive stories were. She pointed out to them that their stories had numerous characters beyond themselves: her parents, his parents, her siblings, her first marriage, his role as an only child—the list was long and varied. The therapist was able to help the couple understand the losses of opportunity their infertility had created. Early in the therapy, she presented these losses as a list of experiences, using a psychoeducational, rather than interpretive, approach. This served to engage the couple's interest in their conflicts, as opposed to focusing on the anger between them.

The therapist talked about Isabel's rift from her family and the ways she had withdrawn from them in an effort to feel mature. She explained the narcissistic blow that Isabel's divorce had caused and the ways in which Paul's narrow definition of generativity was limiting him. In therapy, Isabel and Paul benefited from articulating their reproductive stories to each other; they specified what each needed in order to cope with the trauma. As the therapist helped Isabel understand the ways in which she had retreated from her family, she was able to gently encourage Isabel to consider whether the distance came from them or from her. "You needed to get some distance from your parents in order to feel adult," the therapist remarked. "But you have also ended up missing them and have presumed that they are judging you. Have you considered that they may not feel as critical of you as you have been of them? Perhaps they would be far more supportive than you have been able to give them credit for." When Isabel stepped back and thought about how her parents had tried to connect with her once they got past the initial pain of the divorce and how hurt and left out they had felt when she eloped, she realized that she was projecting her own fears of rejection on to them. With this new perspective, Isabel was able to talk with her family about what she and Paul had been going through. She came to see that although her parents were very involved with their grandchildren, it was not because they were disinterested in her.

Her family turned out to be far more understanding than she had expected. She was especially surprised when her highly religious mother told her that "God gave you this opportunity of medical help, because he wanted you to use it."

Paul, in turn, was able to recognize that continuing the family line was not his responsibility. He learned that there are many different ways to contribute to the next generation, whether they had a child, whether that child was genetically his, or whether they remained child-free. The therapist pointed out that his chosen career as a medical researcher was indeed a way of giving back and helped them both contemplate other meaningful avenues of generativity.

As Paul and Isabel became more comfortable with themselves and confident in their roles as adults, they were able to discuss the options they had to build their family. They decided to try in vitro fertilization (IVF), a decision made easier by Isabel's mother's blessing, and would consider egg donation or adoption if necessary. Although Isabel hoped to have a biological child, she knew how much it meant to both of them to become parents. Furthermore, not only did the couple work out a plan of action, but they also felt more able to share their hurts with each other and felt much closer. They took a break from therapy at that point, promising to return when they were ready to begin their IVF cycle.

SUMMARY

The case of Isabel and Paul illustrates many of the tasks of adult development and the losses of opportunity to achieve these tasks that their infertility created.

Isabel's first failed marriage and then her inability to have a baby left her feeling childlike, unable to feel fully individuated from her family and respected as an autonomous adult. Her career shift from a corporate job to a high school teacher helped enhance her sense of generativity, but it was not the same as having her own child to nurture. Her identity centered on her lifelong wish to become a mother and not solely on her work; without a baby, she felt lost, unsure of how else to consolidate her adult identity. The experience of creating a baby together—one of the most intimate acts in a relationship—was painfully absent from their lives. Both Isabel and Paul felt thwarted in their efforts to maintain a truly intimate relationship. With the marriage strained by the stress of infertility, their longings for a baby with whom they could feel a renewed sense of intimacy were intensified and made them miss the closeness between them even more. As an only child, Paul wanted to continue the family line and provide his parents with a grandchild as an expression of his generativity. Although he valued his work far more than Isabel valued hers, his wish to provide something of himself for the future was nonetheless the focus of his generative fantasies.

Although the developmental tasks of adulthood may not be part of the patient's vocabulary, listening for these themes can alert the mental health practitioner to the profound wounds—and losses of opportunity—that patients bring into therapy. Addressing these issues and bringing them to light can provide a deeper understanding of the enormous psychological damage that results from infertility and reproductive losses.

3

WHEN THE REPRODUCTIVE STORY GOES AWRY: TRAUMA AND LOSS

Because the reproductive story is so deeply ingrained in the sense of self, when it takes an unexpected turn, whether through infertility, premature birth, a pregnancy loss, or, sadly, as often happens, a combination of events, it is a trauma that negatively affects every aspect of a person's life. All too often, patients experience repeated emotional and physical assaults over months or even years, and each menstrual cycle is experienced as yet another failure. As we have discussed, the theory of possible selves focuses not only on the ideal self that people would like to become but also on the selves people are afraid of becoming (Markus & Nurius, 1986). In the case of possible-self-as-parent in the reproductive story, the ideal self would be able to become pregnant easily and have a healthy child, while the feared self might worry about having a miscarriage, infertility, or a child with disabilities. Often, the fears are suppressed and therefore less conscious than the positive ideals. Thus, when the reproductive story goes awry, not only is the possible ideal self negated, but the feared self has become an actuality, adding to the trauma.

WHAT IS REPRODUCTIVE TRAUMA?

A traumatic event, by definition, is exposure to an extremely distressing experience that involves witnessing or undergoing an "actual or threatened death or serious injury, or other threat to one's physical integrity" or to a member of one's family or other close relation (*Diagnostic and Statistical Manual of Mental Disorders* [DSM–IV]; American Psychiatric Association, 1994, p. 424). Whether it is physical or psychological, trauma threatens people's sense of the world as a safe and reliable place and overwhelms their ability to cope. What they have come to expect—their familiar ideas about themselves and their environment—has been severely violated. Reproductive trauma readily fits this definition. "The stressors of infertility [and *all* other negative reproductive events] occur in existential, physical, emotional, and interpersonal realms and may be beyond the average person's usual coping abilities" (Gerrity, 2001, p. 152). Formerly trusting in their bodies, their health, and the tacit belief that pregnancy would be a given, individuals and couples must rethink everything; their dream, represented by their reproductive story, is shattered. The power of this loss is far-reaching: Patients feel their sense of well-being and self-esteem slip away. They are left with a deep narcissistic wound, which erodes the ego, diminishes coping skills, and can lead to disruptions in healthy interpersonal relations.

Unlike other traumas that are one-time occurrences—such as a natural disaster, a serious accident, or a violent assault—it is the chronic nature of infertility and other adverse reproductive events that adds to patients feeling helpless and out of control (Berg & Wilson, 1991). These patients are not unlike soldiers who repeatedly are sent back into battle to conquer the same ever-elusive hill. Indeed, many reproductive clients present with symptoms typical of posttraumatic stress disorder: (a) a continual reliving of the event, (b) a need to avoid stimuli that remind them of the event, and (c) both significant emotional arousal as well as emotional numbing. Their distress is considerable and may also include flashbacks, sleep problems (either insomnia or excessive fatigue), depression, anxiety, difficulty concentrating, irritability, increased startle response, and social isolation (DSM–IV; American Psychiatric Association, 1994; Bartlik, Green, Graf, Sharma, & Melnick, 1997; Born, Phillips, Steiner, & Soares, 2005; Diamond, 2005a, 2005b).

In reproductive cases, reexperiencing the trauma may manifest itself in obsessive thinking. This may be both symptomatic of the traumatized state and also an effort to cope with and master the sense of being overwhelmed by the trauma. Many infertile women, for instance, become fixated on the Internet, searching for diagnoses or the latest technological advances. They may replay conversations with their doctors or have intrusive thoughts about difficult procedures. If a pregnancy loss has occurred, an anniversary date may not only trigger intense emotions but also a reliving of each moment, often with unanswered questions still burning in the patient's mind.

Traumatized people seek to avoid triggers of their traumatic experience (*DSM–IV*; American Psychiatric Association, 1994). For reproductive patients, this occurs when they try to avoid reminders of their childless state, such as seeing pregnant women and babies. Innocuous-seeming situations, like going grocery shopping or dining out, may trigger aversive responses and increase isolation. Avoidance may also occur in a person's reluctance to talk about the reproductive difficulties. This can create conflicts between partners, if one needs to talk and the other needs to not talk. Avoidance may also result in a loss of friendships, especially if peers are having children themselves, and may create feelings of loneliness, despondency, and despair. Love-making may be tarnished, and even feel retraumatizing, by its association with baby-making. Perhaps the most painful and inescapable reminder of all is a woman's monthly menstrual cycle. Even though the need to avoid painful stimuli is great, the reality is that reproductive patients are constantly faced with situations that may retrigger the traumatic response.

The trauma of failed reproductive events is accompanied by multiple losses, including the loss of the reproductive story, that need to be acknowledged and mourned. Because these losses are all encompassing—affecting every aspect of a person's life—symptoms of depression and anxiety are a natural outcome. Depressed patients may report concentration difficulties, sleeping too much or too little, and gaining or losing weight; they may feel lethargic, disinterested, irritable, or impatient; and they may be overly sensitive to criticism. Patients who react with anxiety may feel worried and exceedingly apprehensive, as if around every corner they will encounter yet another obstacle to parenthood. Not every client will experience each and every loss to the same degree, but listening for and reviewing both the obvious and the less apparent losses with patients will make clear the enormity of the trauma they have experienced and will help them understand the depth of their pain. The challenge for clients is to acknowledge that these losses have forever changed them—they are not the person they once were—and to incorporate these losses into a new sense of self (Archer, 1999).

MULTIPLE LOSSES OF REPRODUCTIVE TRAUMA

It can be helpful for the clinician to view these losses through a biopsychosocial lens. Biopsychosocial theory conceptualizes human behavior as the interaction among physical, social, and cognitive or emotional variables (Boyd-Bragadeste, 1998; Gerrity, 2001; Leventhal, 2008). The combination of these various elements serves as a useful theoretical framework for understanding the multiple losses that occur during infertility and other reproductive trauma.

Clearly, *biology* is at the heart of the issue: Clients cannot easily fulfill their hopes and dreams of becoming a biological parent if there are biochemical or anatomical problems. The physical demands of medical tests and procedures can be painful and often require numerous invasive surgeries. Hormonal treatments to enhance ovulation can have negative side effects, such as bloating and abdominal pain, headaches, hot flashes, and/or mood swings. Complications during pregnancy can turn into medical emergencies, requiring bed rest or hospitalization. What one expects to be a "normal" biological process can turn into a health-related nightmare.

Psychologically, the loss of the reproductive story has profound effects on one's sense of self. Patients perceive the failure of their original story as an enormous narcissistic blow. We have seen the most confident and competent people regress to feeling inadequate and insecure in the wake of reproductive problems, both in their personal and professional life. The shame at not being able to achieve their reproductive story as so many others can—and with what seems like great ease—can be devastating and demoralizing. In the face of reproductive trauma, patients can lose sight of who they are. They may feel incompetent, infantilized, and insecure about their identity as a man or woman. Clients may lose a sense of themselves, and they may feel frightened when they don't readily "bounce back" to normal.

Socially, couples and those attempting to be single parents lament that they don't fit in anywhere when their reproductive story does not go as planned. Relationships—with family, friends, and coworkers—can become strained, especially when those close to them are having children. They may feel alienated from their peers, and friendships may disintegrate in the process. They may feel the disappointment of their own parents, as their parents' hopes to become grandparents are delayed. The couple themselves may find their relationship full of tension. They may be arguing more: Not only is their intimate sexual life under fire, they may have to make major health and financial decisions and may have differing opinions on what the next phase of their reproductive story should be. Some may be looking at the use of alternative reproductive technology (such as donor egg or sperm or surrogacy), forcing them to completely rethink their original story and what it means to be a parent. Difficult questions emerge, for example, what is more important, having a genetic connection with a child or having the experience of raising a child, regardless of shared DNA? Or is having a biological child (even if it is through surrogacy) most important? Emotions become intensified when people are under stress, and the couple may find they are angry at each other, or they may blame each other. They may also feel enormously guilty, especially if they feel "at fault" and wonder if their partner will continue to love them if they cannot produce a child.

The following sections describe the multiple losses that may occur. Delineating these losses makes it clear how reproductive loss and infertility affect every aspect of a person's life. And while the reproductive events that patients experience differ, the underlying emotional and psychological impact of the trauma is the same: It is both physical and emotional and represents not only the loss of experience (the focus of this chapter) but also the loss of opportunity to work through the important developmental tasks of adulthood (as discussed in Chapter 2). In talking about the effects of reproductive trauma with clients, mental health professionals can help validate the depth of these losses and their wide-reaching effects. As discussed more fully in Chapter 5, it is only after patients understand the enormous impact that these events have that they can fully mourn.

Loss of the Experience of Pregnancy and Childbirth

An obvious loss for infertility patients or for those who have had a reproductive failure, the inability to become pregnant or to carry a pregnancy to term is nonetheless important to acknowledge. Not only is there no baby to take home, but reproductive trauma also robs couples of the carefree innocence of what they imagined pregnancy would be like. What should have been so easy to achieve—as it appears to be for everyone else—is not. Both men and women may feel as if their body has failed them. And subsequent pregnancies, if they occur, are emotionally challenging, even if all goes well. They are fraught with anxiety and doubt, and, for many, it is only after a baby is born that a couple can let down their guard and feel the previously suppressed emotions.

The loss of the experience of pregnancy and childbirth is painful on many levels. Patients must grieve an experience they may have dreamed of their whole lives. Many women, as soon as they know they are pregnant, shop for maternity clothes; they may even "practice" for how they will look by stuffing pillows into their clothes and admiring their anticipated profile. If a perinatal loss or premature birth has occurred, women physically experience the loss not only of the baby but also of the pregnancy itself. "I loved being pregnant," cried one woman, whose baby was born prematurely at 32 weeks. "Of course, I am happy my baby is okay, but I feel cheated. I loved being pregnant, and I wasn't ready to be done with it."

Furthermore, a woman's sense of identity as truly female is often achieved through pregnancy and childbirth (Leon, 1990). The physicality of a pregnancy is an outward acknowledgement of a woman's sexuality. Miscarriages, which conservative estimates put at approximately 20% of all pregnancies, may represent not only the loss of a child but also the loss of a woman's sense of herself as a fully functioning female. As one woman poignantly told her therapist, "I hate the words used to describe infertility—words like barren or sterile. It makes me feel like some inanimate object, cold and less than human. They talk about the 'fullness of life' as a metaphor for living, but they really are referring to a woman's fecundity and richness. Does that mean that my body is a wasteland?"

Even the most psychologically healthy clients, accomplished in their careers with solid interpersonal relationships, can feel a sense of personal failure in not being able to get pregnant or carry a child to term. Some clients feel that they should be able to overcome infertility, as if conception is something that they just haven't "mastered" yet, rather than understanding it as a medical condition. One of the most important messages that a therapist can convey to both men and women is that *conception is not a skill*. It is not something that people can will to happen. Fertilization of an egg by a sperm is a biochemical reaction, and yet this biological process is so often misconstrued as a psychological one.

Loss of Feeling Healthy and Normal

Because pregnancy is a natural phenomenon, people rarely think of it as a medical condition, but, from a physician's standpoint, all bets are off when a healthy woman becomes, or tries to become, pregnant (B. A. Ourieff, personal communication, December 1985). Although statistically the odds are in her favor that all will go as it should, there is no predicting the course of a pregnancy, if she is able to conceive at all. One of the myths of pregnancy, and a cornerstone of most reproductive stories, is that a woman will be able to get pregnant when and as she chooses, as if this were something totally within her control.

When biology does not cooperate, and pregnancy does not happen as anticipated, people get thrust into a medical arena that does not feel normal or natural, but rather is physically and emotionally painful. According to the American Society for Reproductive Medicine (ASRM), "Infertility is NOT an inconvenience; it is a disease of the reproductive system that impairs the body's ability to perform the basic function of reproduction" (ASRM, 1996–2009). Indeed, infertility, along with other reproductive traumas, is often the first medical crisis that a couple may face in their lives. The identity shift from "physically healthy, normal" to "physically impaired, patient" is another blow to one's sense of self.

With any medical condition, there is a kind of depersonalization that takes place when one becomes a patient, especially if it is for a great length of time. This is often the case for reproductive clients, contributing to their feelings of inadequacy, failure, and diminished self-esteem.

Loss of Control

Giving up control of one's reproductive life and handing it over to a medical team is clearly not a first choice in a person's plans and can be experienced as a painful and frightening loss. Not being able to have a child when and how one had hoped forces one to rethink goals and choices. The irony, of course, is that most people spend a good portion of their adult life trying *not* to get pregnant. Since the development of the Pill in 1960, contraception has made great strides in restricting procreation. The power not to conceive may erroneously lead men and women to believe they have control over reproduction; they have the fantasy that all they need is to stop whatever form of birth control they are using and they will be pregnant the first month they try. Indeed, this is a component of many reproductive stories; even though most people know intellectually that normally it can take several months to conceive, not becoming pregnant on the first try can be a great disappointment.

But the loss of control over the medical piece of reproduction is only one part of the picture. As the following examples illustrate, the feeling of helplessness one experiences can permeate many other facets of one's life, including one's work and relationships. If one is used to setting and achieving goals, feelings of depression, anxiety, and despair may overtake one's sense of competency. Although work can be a much-needed distraction from reproductive struggles, clients often report that they have difficulty concentrating or making decisions at work, leading to even more insecurity and erosion of self-assurance.

Suzanne, a gifted teacher, came to a session one day frazzled and distraught. She launched into a description of her day, lamented that her class was wild, that she could not control them, and concluded that she was a terrible teacher. Suzanne's distress was puzzling to the therapist, as she knew that Suzanne typically found her expertise as a teacher to be a source of pride. As Suzanne gradually calmed down, the therapist was able to say, "You know more about young children than anyone I know, and you know how rambunctious they can become. I wonder if your self-criticism really has more to do with your infertility than with the kids in your class. They may have been unruly, but it is your medical condition that leaves you feeling so out of control." Suzanne's eyes filled with tears as she listened. "I feel so awful about myself, like I can't do anything right, I can't make anything happen correctly." As a way of helping her regain a sense of control, her therapist discussed the need for Suzanne to compartmentalize her struggles with infertility from the rest of her life. By doing so, Suzanne was able to focus on the areas of her life where she did have control and success, thereby mitigating the effects of the reproductive trauma.

Another client, Karen, entered therapy confused and overwhelmed by the various choices, medical and personal, before her. A self-described "planner" by nature, she had chosen to become an accountant because she liked the discipline and sense of order on which her profession was built. She had carefully planned her college curriculum with that goal in mind and had obtained an MBA as well, to give herself the maximum opportunity to be successful. Typical of many individuals (and couples), Karen was used to setting goals and seeing them to fruition, but she had been unable to form an intimate relationship with a partner as she had anticipated, which caused a significant blow to her self-esteem. As she moved through her 30s, she was aware that her biological clock might stop before she found the right partner, and her anxiety increased. Although she was able to track her professional life as planned, her personal life felt out of control. With the help of her therapist, Karen was able to weigh her options: She could risk waiting for the right relationship and hope that she would still be able to have a baby someday, she could freeze her eggs now and thaw them when she was ready to use them (a procedure that to date is costly and not extremely reliable), or she could attempt to have a child as a single woman. Even though Karen has yet to make a decision, simply organizing her choices, making a concrete list, and researching the plusses and minuses of each possibility have allowed her to reclaim control over her reproductive story.

Self-Blame and Shame

The early psychoanalytic explanation of pregnancy loss and infertility was based on psychogenic theory: the idea that psychological disorders are a result of unresolved, and often unconscious, conflicts (Burns & Covington, 2000). This theory contended that pregnancy failures that were not founded on clear medical pathology were caused by emotional factors. In particular, it was thought that a woman's ambivalence *about* becoming a mother—her unresolved issues and internal tensions with her own mother—was the cause of her procreative problems (Benedek, 1952; Deutsch, 1945; Leon, 1990). With the enormous advances in the medical understanding of these reproductive events, we now know that, in most cases, the psychogenic theory of reproductive loss is not accurate. Rather than viewing psychological disorders as the *cause* of infertility or miscarriage, it is now widely believed that they occur as an *effect* of not being able to have a child (Leon, 1990). As noted, the process of being diagnosed and treated is overwhelming; it depletes one's coping reserves and can be the cause of psychological problems, instead of the other way around (Andrews, Abbey, & Halman, 1991; Blenner, 1992).

Although most clients reject the notion that their reproductive problems are because of unresolved psychological conflicts, the tendency to blame themselves for some aspect of the loss is almost universal. The questions: "Why me?" or "What did we do wrong?" frequently pop up in the clinical setting. Although not always rational, and almost always inaccurate, these clients find it more reassuring to blame themselves for their reproductive crisis, rather than believing it to be a random event. Sometimes patients look to the past to find some justification for their current trauma. They may worry about former relationships and conflicts. Indeed, it is not uncommon for patients to blame their infertility or pregnancy loss on past indiscretions (Berg, Wilson, & Weingartner, 1991; Mahlstedt, 1994; Mazor, 1984). They deduce that it must have been the partying they had done in college, or perhaps it was the premarital sex that they suddenly feel guilty about. In addition, they may fear that ambivalent or anxious thoughts about having a child—as normal as it is to have these thoughts—may affect their ability to conceive. Rationally, they may understand that thinking cannot prevent a pregnancy (if this were the case, there would be no need for birth control!), but, emotionally, they may feel guilty for even questioning themselves.

A previous unwanted pregnancy, whether the person relinquished the baby for adoption or had an abortion, is a vital issue that may reemerge as a client contends with his or her current reproductive trauma and loss. Even if the sentiments surrounding the unwanted pregnancy were resolved and previously put to rest, thoughts and feelings may resurface. People have a tendency to rewrite history in their efforts to understand their current reproductive difficulties; they may revisit a past decision and conclude they had made a terrible mistake, even if it was absolutely the right choice at the time. Both men and women may feel that they have lost their only chance at parenthood or that they are being punished for their previous decision, even if it was not experienced that way originally. One woman, who had an abortion at 19, did not regret it but could not help but think about it: "If I had to do it over again, I would have made the same choice now as then. But sometimes I wonder if that was my only chance at becoming a mom." As we discuss in Chapter 4, it is important for the therapist to inquire about a client's reproductive history to explore these feelings.

Are We Parents or Not?

A medical procedure such as in vitro fertilization (IVF) allows individuals and couples a remarkable view into the biological processes of reproduction. Because clients literally can see their "babies" when they are just a few cells old, the attachment to their potential child(ren) and their own identity as parents begins far sooner than any eventual pregnancy test. This is a loss that often goes unrecognized—the sense of self as "a little bit pregnant" when embryos are developing—even before implantation. As one woman said in her efforts to comfort herself after a failed IVF cycle, "At least I was a mom for a few days."

The impact on one's identity is that much more intense if a miscarriage, stillbirth, or other perinatal loss occurs. Paula was 30 weeks along when she lost her daughter. "I went to bed feeling her moving, but as soon as I woke up I knew something was wrong." By the time she arrived in the emergency room, there was no heartbeat. There had been no prior indications that anything was amiss; in fact, Paula had seen her obstetrician only 3 days before. She was induced, and 8 hr later delivered her baby. "We held her for hours; she was perfect in every way, except she wasn't breathing, she wasn't crying . . . and she never will. I kept thinking, 'I'm a mom, but how can I be a mom if my baby is not here?'"

Paula's questioning of her role as a mother points to the profound effect reproductive loss has on one's parental identity. The sense of failure is massive, equal only to the feelings of guilt. The reasoning behind the self-blame goes something like this: If I became a parent, only to have my baby die, then I must be a terrible parent. The "if-only's" that mothers ruminate on can fill an entire book: if only I hadn't taken such a long walk; if only I hadn't painted the baby's room; if only I had woken up earlier, paged the doctor, gone to the hospital sooner, and on and on. Again, rationally, these women know they did nothing to harm their baby, but emotionally they feel they *must* have done something wrong. As one woman movingly put it, "I feel as if I somehow poisoned my baby, that there must have been something bad inside me. How can I ever consider getting pregnant again? This baby is gone, but the badness is still there."

With a reproductive loss, one's sense of identity as parent gets challenged in ordinary, everyday interchanges with strangers. How does one respond to the query, "Do you have any children?" The struggle with how to answer that question goes right to the heart of one's sense of identity. To answer "Yes, but my baby died" is difficult, to say the least, and may not feel appropriate depending on the situation, but to reply "No" may feel disrespectful to their child and denies an important part of themselves. The clinician can help guide the client through these awkward social situations, practicing possible responses and giving "permission" to respond in the way that feels most suitable. It can help clients to know that, even if outwardly they deny their loss, they can still acknowledge and honor their child to themselves.

Loss of One's Sense of Self

If a patient had a broken arm or had to wear glasses, his or her reaction might be: A part of me needs mending, or a part of my body is weak. The client would go about correcting the problem, without feeling like something was wrong with his or her core identity. But with a reproductive trauma, patients tend to respond with statements that encompass the entire self. They are more likely to say, "I am infertile" rather than, "There is something wrong with a part of my body." It is this connection, between one's reproductive organs and one's identity, that makes one feel like a failure (Jaffe, Diamond, & Diamond, 2005).

The association between one's reproductive system and one's self-perception is powerful for both men and women, albeit in different ways. The differences in gender reactions are discussed in greater detail in Chapter 6, but the losses involved for each are significant. For a man, infertility threatens his sense of virility, his sense of manliness. His ego may take a hit, especially if he compares himself with other men; he may feel less effectual, more insecure, and consequently may doubt his abilities, not just in having a child but in other aspects of his life. Although parenthood may be greatly desired by both men and women, the idea of becoming a parent is less central to a man's sense of self. A man's role in the family has evolved over time, and, historically speaking, his identity has been more strongly defined by his social role of employment outside of the home (Berg, Wilson, & Weingartner, 1991).

In contrast, becoming a mother is often central to a woman's identity (Kittrell, 1998; Levinson, 1978). When a woman reflects on her reproductive story, she will do so in great detail, revealing the innermost dreams and definition of herself. Whether as a result of societal expectations or an innate biological drive, most women consider motherhood a major life goal. Her unique ability to bear a child establishes her sexuality, defines her as an adult woman, and sets her apart from men; indeed, sometimes it is only through childbearing that a woman can fully understand how her hidden internal reproductive organs actually work. Whereas men have been socialized to work and derive their self-view from vocational goals, women may view their professional life as something that competes with their commitment to family life or that is an adjunct to raising children (Kittrell, 1998; Roberts & Newton, 1987). Although women's choices tend to be much broader in current society than in the past, a woman's sense of self is often defined more by her role as mother than by her title at work. Because of this, when motherhood is denied either by infertility or by other pregnancy loss, the narcissistic injury can be profound. Not only is her sense of femininity diminished, but the failure to live up to cultural expectations may cast enormous doubts on her self-definition, leading to acute feelings of worthlessness and inadequacy (Berg et al., 1991; Burns, 2000; Leon, 1990).

Loss of a Sense of Belonging

Individuals and couples who struggle with infertility or perinatal loss often feel painfully alienated from friends or family who are pregnant or who have small children. One patient described herself as being on one side of a fence while the entire fertile world seemed like it was on the other. Another remarked that, "It was just a few years ago when all of my friends were getting married. And then it started—one by one—everyone was having kids. I felt more and more out of sync with them; I no longer belonged." Paradoxically, clients may also feel as if they don't fit in with single friends or other child-free couples. They may have made the psychological shift in their parental identity, without having the physical reality of having a family. They may perceive others who are childfree as having the luxury of choice; this can engender envy as much as the pregnancies of others can.

As such, reproductive clients may feel an enormous sense of isolation. Understandably, they may withdraw to protect themselves from overexposure to others who are pregnant, which inevitably reminds them of what is missing in their life. It can be extraordinarily painful, for example, to attend baby showers or other events focused on children. If people choose to attend, they may feel miserable; if they don't, they may feel as if they are not good, supportive friends. Either way, they struggle. Likewise, at the workplace, they are often faced with determining how to handle their feelings if a coworker brings in photos of his or her newborn. Clients can try to put on a good front and congratulate the new mom or dad, but, inside, they may feel like crying. These no-win situations add to the despair and isolation individuals and couples feel.

Those struggling with reproductive difficulties may also feel like misfits within their own family. Family gatherings, such as birthday parties or holiday celebrations, are often geared toward children, again drawing attention to what is absent for them. The focus on family also highlights the fact that the reproductive story is multigenerational; would-be-grandparents may feel as if their story has also gone awry. Their desire to have grandchildren can feel like added pressure to the childless, sometimes with overt coaxing but often addressed in more subtle ways. Psychologically, it may pain them deeply that their own child, their baby, is struggling to create a family, and they may feel at a loss to know how to help and support their son or daughter. Guilt over their own ability to have children and/or unhealthy competitive issues with their own child or children may emerge, or they may wonder if somehow they are to blame, passing on a biological malfunction. Furthermore, their child's experience may reevoke memories of their own reproductive traumas that they had not shared with anyone for decades. Interestingly, the older generation may experience their own social pressures as well: As *their* peer group has gained grandchildren, they may feel out of place, just as their infertile offspring do. The reactions that would-be-grandparents have can be yet another component to how their children cope.

Additionally, clients are often exposed to off-putting comments that people make in misguided efforts to be of comfort. Remarks like, "You're young, you can have another" or "It was for the best" or "The fun is in the trying" can leave those who are grief-stricken feeling more misunderstood than ever. These comments may be well intentioned, but they minimize clients' physical and psychological pain. It can be very useful for the therapist to help patients think of responses to such comments, that they "can keep in their back pockets," so to speak, so that they are not caught off-guard when confronted by well-meaning but ignorant people. Kindly letting someone know that having a miscarriage, for instance, is not "for the best" not only helps empower patients in these very awkward moments but also serves to educate others that their "support" actually hurts.

In this context, therapists can—and should—encourage clients to consider joining a support group. It is important for people to be with others who truly understand and who can identify with their pain and trauma. As discussed more thoroughly in Chapter 9, support groups, whether face-to-face or online, can feel like lifeboats for those who are feeling adrift and disconnected from others. They can provide much-needed comfort and counter the sense of isolation.

Loss of Closeness With One's Partner

As discussed in Chapter 2, a significant adult developmental step is the formation of an intimate mature relationship outside the family of origin. This sense of deep connection can be further enhanced by having a baby and may be at risk when a couple experiences reproductive problems. For many couples, reproductive trauma is a bonding experience. The couple may pull together as they commit to working toward a common goal, and they are able to provide sustaining support to each other throughout the ordeal. This is not the case for all couples, however, and many find themselves in the midst of relational stress when faced with a reproductive crisis. Even the best of relationships bow under the strain of adverse reproductive events—not surprising, given the intensity of medical treatments, raging hormones, and enormous financial obligations, all combined with underlying anger and grief.

Anger can be a potent contributor to the struggles in the relationship. It's normal for clients to feel angry when they've had a reproductive loss, anger being a typical reaction to grief and loss. Couples may get frustrated with their doctor and medical staff, may feel infuriated with friends or family, may feel spiritually depleted and angry with God, may turn their anger inward, or, as so often happens, they may take their disappointments out on each other. Not surprising, it's the person they feel closest to who may bear the brunt of all their negative feelings. When couples can identify what they are really angry about—that is, not being able to have a baby—they usually can put their feelings about each other back into perspective.

There are times, however, when a couple will just not see eye to eye on how to handle their loss. Because each person grieves in their own time and in their own way (as discussed more thoroughly in Chapters 5 and 6), their differences may cause friction in the relationship. It is often the case, for example, that one person will feel more ready to move forward than the other or will want to move forward in a different way: She may be ready to explore adoption, whereas he may be desperate to try another IVF. When left unchecked, the frustration and loss of control over not being able to have a baby can get transferred to issues of power and control between them. They may bicker or fight over otherwise innocuous decisions, like where to go for dinner or what chairs to buy, and skirt the real issue at hand. It is helpful for the therapist to point out this pattern and to teach clients how to negotiate with each other and compromise in ways that satisfy both their needs as much as possible. Maybe, for example, *she* will agree to one more round of IVF, out of respect for *his* needs, after which they will pursue their family through adoption, as *she* wishes. It can be helpful to remind the couple that they have been able to problem-solve effectively many other times before in their relationship and to remind them of all the decisions they have already made as a team, be it where to go for vacation or what house to buy. This not only reminds the couple of the importance of compromise, but it also brings them back in touch with the strengths of their relationship, qualities that may have become mired in the angst of the current struggles. Whatever the resolution of any given issue, the task at hand is to realign the couple to their sense of being a team.

Loss of Sexual Intimacy and Privacy

The sexual component of a relationship is a complex mixture of the physical, social, and emotional needs of the couple (Burns, 2000). As discussed in greater detail in Chapter 6, a couple's initial efforts to have a baby often increase their passion for each other, but over time, infertility causes the regimentation of sex, and desire tends to dampen. With infertility, what was once the most romantic, intimate, and pleasurable of acts falls under the scrutiny of medical professionals and comes laden with thermometers, kits, timetables, and shots. Spontaneity is a bygone pleasure: When ovulation occurs, sex is required, whether either partner is in the mood or not. The act of making a baby, which should have happened in privacy, may now take place in a sterile hospital room or in a doctor's office under the glare of fluorescent lights. The pressure to perform may create its own set of problems—avoidance or erectile dysfunction—which, in turn, may add to the fertility problem. With a previous pregnancy failure, the sexual act may become even more emotionally complex. There is, of course, the hope that a new pregnancy will occur, but at the same time, the memory of the loss and the possibility of another can create excessive anxiety in both partners, again detracting from sexual desire and adding to performance pressures.

The effect of reproductive trauma on a couple's sexual relationship has potentially far-reaching implications as well. At the individual level, loss of sexual desire or potency can erode a person's sense of him- or herself as fully masculine or feminine. It can leave a person feeling childlike and regressed and can cause another blow to self-esteem, already weakened by the reproductive failures. It can feel as if there is yet something else wrong with them, something abnormal, that sets them apart. Additionally, a wedge can develop between members of the couple, as each person's approach or avoidance is potentially misinterpreted by the other. Traumatized couples with low self-esteem may not allow themselves the pleasure of intimate lovemaking, even after they have stopped "trying," because they may not feel deserving. Finally, as previously mentioned, when lovemaking becomes inextricably tied up with baby-making, what once had been intimate and joyful may now serve as a constant reminder of what they were not able to create.

Loss of Financial Freedom

Using assisted reproductive technologies (ART) can be exorbitantly expensive. The average cost of a single IVF cycle in the United States is $12,400 (ASRM, 1996–2009); some physicians suggest limiting IVF to three trials, but many couples opt for more, incurring huge debts. Although most insurance plans do not cover the procedure itself, some will pay for medications and/or monitoring. To date, only 14 states have laws requiring insurance companies to cover at least some of the expenses of IVF, but the scope of the legislation varies greatly from state to state (ASRM, 2000–2009). The cost of a donor egg or embryo cycle can range from $15,000 to $30,000; included in this is the cost of compensation for the donor, which can vary between $5,000 and $15,000. However, if it is a repeat donor, or if she is considered "exceptional," her fees may be even higher (Egg Donation Inc., 2008). Fees for adoption, either domestic or international, generally range from $15,000 to $30,000 (Salzer, 2000).

It is not uncommon for an individual or couple to find themselves in the position of wanting to adopt after several failed IVF cycles. If they can afford to pursue adoption at that point, they may find themselves having spent upward of $100,000 in their efforts to create a family. The financial constraint this creates is enormous. Many must borrow money to finance their treatment or adoption; some may ask parents or other family members, opening themselves up for what could be a host of complicated dynamics; others may borrow against a house or use savings or retirement funds that would have been otherwise directed; still others may have to make treatment decisions or stop treatment altogether, according to their financial situation. All of these

circumstances also increase the risk of disrupting the couple's adult developmental track by placing them in regressed, dependent positions or by the
experience of moving backward professionally and financially in the face of
the economic strain. Under the best of circumstances, money matters are
often the basis for relational discord; each member of the couple may have
different views on spending and saving, disagreeing on what is a priority.
When the financial burdens of reproductive technology or adoption are added
into the mix, it's no wonder couples feel so distraught. Like adding insult to
injury, it's especially hurtful when other couples, who are able to create their
family the "old-fashioned way," do so without any financial hardship.

Loss of Trust in the World

Perhaps one of the most disconcerting feelings brought on by these
upsetting reproductive trials is the loss of faith in the world and how it works.
Infertility and pregnancy loss are truly life-altering events, shaking the very
foundations of one's belief system. Both trust in oneself as competent and
trust in the world as just and fair are undermined. It is not uncommon for
deep and painful existential questions to arise concerning the meaning and
purpose of life.

Religious beliefs and questions about God often become part of the
clinical arena. Clinically, the therapist must allow the client freedom to
explore these feelings, not make assumptions, and, as discussed further in
Chapter 8, remain neutral in terms of his or her own personal belief system.
Some patients, for example, may give meaning to their trauma by their belief
that God has given them this challenging situation in life for a reason: There
is a lesson to be learned from it or a larger plan in store for them. For these
clients, the idea that everything has a purpose, that their infertility or loss is
not just some random, meaningless event, brings them comfort. They take
solace and find strength by putting their lives and the outcome of their trauma
in God's hands. But for others, doubts about God and religion develop, which
can be very unsettling. People wonder, "Why me? What have I done to deserve
this?"—as if their reproductive loss was a punishment for some wrongdoing.
They may question or feel abandoned by God; the anger they feel may add to
feelings of guilt and shame. They may miss the feeling of solidity that their
faith once provided. One patient, who had suffered for years from her doubts
in God, visited a priest while on vacation. She came home with a renewed
sense of faith and noted that she felt whole again. "I realized that God had
not abandoned me, but that I had abandoned God, and I could choose to
reconnect with Him. I feel so much less alone and more in control now."

It may also be that the desire to pursue medical treatments, such as
IVF, is in direct conflict with the tenets of one's religion. Although having

children may be a fundamental value in all religions and cultures, some religious institutions decry reproductive technology as unnatural. It is important for therapists to be aware of the conflicts this situation may create in patients and be sensitive to the discrepant feelings it elicits. Clients may feel that if they pursue ART they are abandoning their faith; they may also worry that their place of worship will abandon or judge them or their child. Just as with cultural stereotypes, the mental health professional should not make assumptions on the basis of religious orientation but should explore the meaning of spiritual beliefs for each individual or couple.

SUMMARY

The focus of this chapter has been on the losses experienced by couples faced with infertility or other reproductive trauma—and the far-reaching impact of these losses. These multiple losses affect the individual's sense of self; the relationship with his or her partner; relationships with family, friends, and coworkers; and feelings about the meaning of life itself. Couples are often unprepared for the enormous toll adverse reproductive events can have. In their need to protect themselves from their pain and "get back to normal," they may minimize these losses and deny the intensity of their feelings when their reproductive story goes awry, leading to symptomatic reactions. Bringing these losses into consciousness helps to validate the experience. As discussed in Chapter 5, clinicians play a vital role in facilitating grieving, by helping patients label and acknowledge these multiple layers of loss.

II

COUNSELING THE
REPRODUCTIVE PATIENT

4

TECHNIQUES OF ASSESSMENT
AND TREATMENT

Before delving into the methods of assessment and treatment of reproductive patients, a few caveats are in order. First, it is important to realize that, despite their great need for empathy and support, reproductive patients are sometimes reluctant to seek therapy and often feel a sense of shame at doing so. Because infertility and pregnancy loss are so interconnected with one's sense of self, patients may already feel like failures as they shift from "normal" to "reproductive patient." By now narcissistically wounded by not being able to conceive without medical help, patients can feel as if psychotherapy is yet another defeat. The need for psychological services translates into yet something else they can't do on their own and must have help with. The therapist must never forget that these patients are extremely vulnerable and have come to therapy because they are feeling desperate. It is important to label their experience as a trauma, even without knowing the details, and to emphasize the strength they have shown in coming in. They may need to be reassured that the therapist is there to provide support and understanding and to help them during this extraordinarily difficult time of their life. It is important to dispel the belief that there is "something wrong with them for needing therapy." Therapy needs to be normalized as something very appropriate for

71

traumatized people and viewed as part of their self-care. These simple comments can immediately feel like salve on the narcissistic wounds they have suffered.

Therapy with reproductive patients is different, at least at the outset, from therapy with neurotic patients who seek long-term psychotherapy. Unlike people who seek therapeutic help for other issues, these clients tend to be focused specifically on reproductive problems. They do not necessarily enter therapy to deal with family of origin conflicts or to make fundamental changes to their personality, and, in fact, it may be counterproductive to do so, given the enormous duress they are under. Although other concerns naturally seep into the therapy, more often than not the issues tend to be directly or indirectly related to procreation, loss, the trauma of medical treatment, and their sense of self as parent. Invariably, themes related to their relationships with their parents emerge, as part of their reproductive story and parental identity.

Second, as we embark on a discussion of assessment and treatment, it is important to remember that therapy with reproductive patients does not usually unfold in the same way as therapy with other kinds of patients. "Assessment" may take many sessions to complete, and "treatment" really begins with the first session.

Patients come to therapy in crisis, and early treatment may resemble crisis intervention work more than psychotherapy. Remember that by the time an individual or couple seeks psychotherapy for a reproductive trauma or loss, they are most likely feeling depleted and demoralized—physically, emotionally, and financially. They may have been through any number of tests, procedures, and/or surgeries; may have experienced or witnessed a medical emergency; and may have spent enormous sums of money as well as time in pursuit of their dream. They may be feeling fragile, their defenses brittle and worn. They may feel isolated and alienated, because infertility and pregnancy loss are often unrecognized by society (Shapiro, 1988) and there are no socially sanctioned rituals through which to share the grief. With grief viewed as a taboo that should not be discussed, couples feel alone with their loss.

As noted in Chapter 2, pregnancy under normal conditions can be considered a developmental upheaval (Benedek, 1959; Bibring, 1959; Colarusso, 1990; Leon, 1990). A reproductive crisis, which is commonly prolonged, within the normal developmental challenges of the transition to parenthood, is often what causes individuals or couples to seek out psychological help (Applegarth, 2000). They may worry that therapy will not help them, that they will never feel differently than they do now. As such, the first interventions may consist of asking them to tell the therapist what has just happened. They will benefit from the therapist acknowledging their experience as a trauma and commending them for coming in. They may also benefit from reassurance that patients find this kind of therapy very helpful and that they *can* work through these difficulties.

72   REPRODUCTIVE TRAUMA

As we discuss other aspects of assessment, including the reproductive story, one must keep in mind that this is not a linear process of history gathering the way it is for other patients. There are so many biological, psychological, and social aspects to reproductive trauma that patients may need to discuss any one of these at any time; it is imperative that the therapist remain flexible and supportive and be truly willing to "take the patient where he or she is at" to avoid alienating them or leaving them feeling as if "you just don't get it." In essence, the "course of therapy" with reproductive patients would be more appropriately called "layers of therapy," with any given layer coming to the surface at any time.

Patients dealing with infertility and/or pregnancy loss may seek psychological treatment and support at any point in their struggle. However, from our clinical observation, there appear to be key times when individuals and/or couples are more likely to reach out for help than not:

- at the time of diagnosis or first visit to a reproductive endocrinologist,
- during stressful in vitro fertilization (IVF) procedures,
- after multiple IVF attempts and failures or when facing yet another cycle,
- after a pregnancy loss,
- on reaching a crossroads in deciding about other available family-building options,
- when couples differ in these choices, and
- if they are planning to use third-party reproductive technology (using donors or surrogates).

In each of these situations, a thorough assessment is necessary to fully understand the needs and goals for each person in the dyad. As emphasized previously, it is important to note that, although in many settings an initial evaluation is completed in one session, with reproductive patients this process is likely to require several sessions or even months because of some of the special needs of these patients. Some issues may need to be addressed early in treatment, issues that may not come up so soon in other kinds of therapies. This chapter provides a clinical overview and checklist to assist the mental health provider in evaluating the reproductive client.

Although insight and understanding remain the primary therapeutic tools in working with reproductive patients, traditional techniques often need to give way to a more flexible, supportive, interactive style. Insight that is provided in the context of psychoeducation and problem solving is often most effective. Because patients present with a wide variety of symptoms that overlap with multiple diagnoses, no single treatment plan is adequate to address their needs. An eclectic style to treating reproductive patients is therefore recommended, combining psychoeducation with various other methods to reduce emotional distress, augment self-esteem, allow for catharsis, and increase communication and understanding between the patient and his or her partner. These include cognitive therapy, psychodynamic therapy, self-psychology, grief work, exposure, and supportive therapy for either the individual or couple.

This chapter also discusses typical diagnoses for this population. Many patients exhibit classic symptoms of depression and/or anxiety as both women and men cope with their grief. Anger, often overlooked as a symptom of depression, is a common reaction, especially among men, and can be quite unsettling to the individual or couple. It is also not unusual for obsessive traits or behaviors to emerge during infertility treatment. In addition, characteristics of posttraumatic stress disorder, including flashbacks and feelings of dissociation and avoidance, are common. It is essential for the clinician to distinguish between prior "normal" functioning and current symptoms brought on by elevated levels of distress.

THE INITIAL APPOINTMENT

No matter what one's theoretical framework, the initial session(s) of a reproductive case should be devoted to hearing the patient's current story and concerns. The more general aspects of the patient's background and history may not be explored until several sessions have been held. This delay can make some therapists feel as if they are not doing a thorough job, but they need to remember that these patients arrive in a traumatized state. Often, the early sessions of a reproductive patient unfold more like crisis interventions or emergency room debriefings, rather than the methodical, orderly intake process of patients presenting with neurotic problems. Reproductive patients do not enter therapy to make fundamental changes to their personality; rather, they come to repair their sense of self and return to feeling whole again (Leon, 1996). Their stories are painful to hear; the loss of a baby, whether that child is full term or merely a blastocyst, is devastating, and the intensity of the emotions parents feel can be overpowering.

Often, clients are encouraged by well-meaning relatives not to talk about or dwell on their pain; they are advised to "put it behind you and move on." But patients have a need to address their stories and their feelings—over and over again. By listening to the details of the trauma without judgment, the therapist gives permission to air these negative thoughts and feelings and allows the client to feel understood. As basic as this may seem to seasoned therapists, there have been many angry reports from patients whose initial contact had been with a health care provider untrained in treating the emotional aspects of reproductive loss. One such case occurred soon after a couple had lost their premature son. The therapist they saw had great empathy for their loss but then continued with a routine exploration of their family background and relationship history. The couple left feeling unheard, misunderstood, and more at a loss than when they started. Indeed, a major concern of reproductive clients seeking treatment is that their health care provider does not understand the full extent of what they are going through (Hart, 2002).

Infertility and/or pregnancy loss produces a huge psychological crisis for patients. It is important to remember that these patients are already in a sensitized state, given the normal psychological adjustments necessary to be made in preparation for pregnancy (Leon, 1990). So much feels out of control; they have been thrown an unexpected left hook that hits at their very core. They often feel as if they are going crazy; all they can dwell on is the quest to have a family. Knowing what is normal under these abnormal conditions can be hugely helpful to them. Having a therapist normalize and validate their feelings brings an enormous sense of relief. In our practices, we have witnessed countless sighs of relief from patients as they recognize that their thoughts and feelings are normal, even if they seem irrational to friends and family—or even to themselves; they need to know that their reactions are to be expected, given the blow to their ego and loss of so many elements of their reproductive story. Acknowledging this in the initial appointments helps to release the patient's anxiety, reduce their stress, and ameliorate feelings of isolation.

USING THE REPRODUCTIVE STORY AS AN ASSESSMENT AID

Once the presenting crisis has been processed, it can be very helpful to introduce the concept of the reproductive story early on in treatment; this can help address several issues at once. Having patients talk about what they had hoped for and what they anticipated pregnancy and parenthood would be like illuminates the full extent of what they have lost. Only once the multiple layers of losses are recognized as such can grieving take place. When the underlying meaning of these losses is discussed, it not only provides vital information to the therapist but also facilitates open dialogue between the couple.

"This Was Not the Way It Was Supposed To Be"

This is the message that clients cry as they express their pain and anguish. Once they have been able to release some of the emotions about the immediate trauma, having patients talk about their original reproductive story—how it *was* supposed to be—can help them identify the multiple losses they have incurred. When patients tell their story, the therapist can gain knowledge of the salient features of the patient's loss. It gives the clinician a working model of the meaning of pregnancy and parenthood for each individual patient. Rachel, for example, a 32-year-old woman who had suffered multiple miscarriages, felt like a complete failure. "All the women in my family got pregnant so easily," she lamented. "I am the last one of the cousins not to be a parent yet. And when we were all young, I was the one who always took care of the other kids. My nickname was 'little mommy'." A portion of Rachel's definition of self is as the "little mommy" of her peers in the family. Not only had she struggled with miscarriages but she had also lost feeling special in the family hierarchy. For the clinician, this knowledge can help him or her formulate a treatment plan, in this case focusing on grief work and the use of cognitive therapy as a reparative effort necessary to rebuild the client's sense of self.

Gathering History

When patients reflect on how they thought parenthood should have happened, it can help them put their loss into the context of their life and thus serve as a means for the clinician to collect relevant family history. Rachel, for example, went on to talk about her family. "My grandparents were Holocaust survivors," she explained. "My parents, my aunts, and my uncles have always talked about how important it is to have children, to honor those who were lost and to replenish our people. Every time I miscarry, I feel like I have let them down."

Inquiring about other times the reproductive story may have gone awry is another way of gathering personal history. Again, this may or may not be appropriate until initial sessions are past, but eventually this can open the door to discussion of relationship history, promiscuity, and sexual functioning. Patients often will not readily offer this information, especially about previous sexual experiences, pregnancies, or pregnancy terminations. The therapist must ask these questions gently, but by putting them in the context of understanding the reproductive story, patients often feel more at ease, indeed, relieved, to talk about them. For example, Sandra and Jack came in for supportive therapy during a pregnancy that was complicated due to a cardiac anomaly in the fetus, which it was unlikely to survive. This was the couple's fourth child, and they felt determined to continue the pregnancy, despite recommendations against it from doctors and family members. As the therapist explored this, she began by acknowledging the couple's fortitude and courage in the face of this trauma. As the layers of therapy unfolded, she was able to ask about prior times when they were challenged like this. It turns out that Sandra and Jack, who had been together since high school, had conceived when she was 17. Their parents "forced them to have an abortion," something neither of them believed in. They had each carried this unresolved grief for all those years, never talking about it until it came up in treatment. The therapist asked if they thought their wish to have a large family was to help them make up for their abortion. She wondered with them if each child, including this one, had been experienced as a replacement for the baby they aborted, an "evening up of number of pregnancies and number of children." This effort had gone well until now: With a threatened pregnancy, they risked the loss of another child.

This dynamically oriented therapy allowed Sandra and Jack to work through some of their earlier grief, and with the insight they gained, they were able to consider the medical status of the current pregnancy more realistically. The couple became more open to terminating the pregnancy, although they agreed to one more consultation before making the final decision. They met with a specialist who was developing a new procedure involving intrauterine surgery to correct cardiac problems. Although frightened, Sandra and Jack chose to have the surgery, which, fortunately, resulted in their baby being born healthy. With this experience, and with what they learned in therapy, however, the couple were finally able to lay to rest their traumatic abortion and to enjoy their children in their own right.

Facilitating Dialogue With One's Partner

In couples therapy, the reproductive story can serve as a catalyst to promote dialogue with one's partner. Over time, as each individual shares his or her original reproductive story, the understanding of the meaning of the failure deepens. It is especially important for the identified patient to express his or her experience of the trauma itself, as well as feelings of shame, sadness, and fear. The infertile member of the couple may be afraid that the fertile partner will leave to create a family elsewhere (Klock, 2006). They may be plagued with horrifying visual images or what they feel are unacceptable emotions. These fears are often unvoiced and create a great deal of anxiety, especially because the fears are usually unfounded in reality. It can sometimes help if the therapist is proactive in naming some of these fears in a didactic way, not unlike using displacement when working with kids or adolescents; it gives patients "permission" to feel whatever they are feeling and renders it less unspeakable. The therapist can use phrases such as "Often people who have gone through this kind of trauma will worry that their partner will blame them . . . that they should be ashamed . . . that they are to blame . . . that they have nightmares . . . that they cannot tell anyone the details of their physical experience because they worry that it is too awful for someone (even a therapist) to hear." The therapist can say, "Whether or not you feel these things, it is important to know that such feelings are normal." When couples share their feelings and the personal meaning of failure and responsibility, the therapist can help them recognize their insecurities and enable them to support each other.

Because the reproductive story is unique to each member of the dyad, knowing how the other feels about creating a family—or not—is essential. When partners do not share the same reproductive goals, for example, they may feel they must choose between their relationship and the desire to have a child. Cultural and religious conflicts may emerge, or financial and pragmatic concerns may cause one person to question continued treatment or other reproductive decisions. The goal in these cases is for a deeper understanding of each other's needs and, if possible, to come to a compromise.

Joe and Maggie, a couple in their mid-30s, had delayed family building so that they could enjoy some time as a couple. Joe had been ambivalent about having kids at all but agreed when Maggie expressed her intense wish to have a child. Maggie was devastated when she was told that the age of her eggs was likely the cause of their infertility. She became eager to pursue every possible means of having a baby, including using an egg donor. Joe reluctantly agreed to intrauterine insemination (IUI)—even though their chances of conception using this method were very low—but drew an absolute line in the sand at any more invasive interventions, creating enormous conflict between them. He was completely opposed to egg donation, although Maggie thought it was a great solution; she was not at all concerned that a child conceived this way would not feel like her own.

The therapist was puzzled by Joe's absolute refusal to consider other treatments, even though he saw how important it was to his wife. She finally persuaded Joe to come in for some individual sessions to try to understand why he felt the way he did. Over a number of sessions, Joe, who was the eldest of his three siblings, was able to reveal that his own parents had suffered numerous reproductive traumas, including the loss of twins, multiple miscarriages, and medical emergencies, and that there were long stretches of time in which he remembered his mother bedridden and very sad. He was absolutely terrified of pregnancy, birth, and reproductive loss. He had overcome this to the extent that he agreed to try to have a biological child with his wife, but he would not take on the risks he had observed as a youngster, for a child that would not be "their own." The therapist encouraged Joe to explain his feelings to his wife—he had never told anyone about this—and he did so in a joint session. When Maggie understood why her husband was so resistant, she was able to feel compassion rather than anger toward him. As she became less critical, he became less frightened and rigid, and they were able to decide on a course of action that was right for them.

This kind of dialogue sometimes occurs even if only one member of the couple is in therapy. Often, the patient will go home and talk about the reproductive story with his or her partner. It can draw them closer and engage the nonparticipating person in the therapy. This is the kind of ripple effect that can occur, whereby the whole family is helped even if only one person is in treatment.

Making Decisions About the Future

As Joe and Maggie so aptly demonstrated, knowing where and why one's reproductive story diverges from one's partner can be key in exploring future alternative reproductive options. When mental health practitioners understand what drives their clients' feelings about creating a family—and the various ways in which it might come about—they can promote negotiation between the partners, and compromise becomes a possibility. Understanding the internal dynamics of each person's story allows the therapist to address the stumbling blocks that are preventing them from moving forward.

FURTHER FACTORS IN ASSESSMENT AND TREATMENT

There are additional important details that should be addressed early on in the treatment of these cases. The following topics present a brief description of areas that should be investigated with new patients, but the timing and order in which they come up will vary according to the patient's needs.

Medical History

The medical experience of infertility and reproductive loss is integral to the therapy. For many patients, the traumas of the medical procedures and/or hospital stays are as vivid to them as they recount them in the therapist's office as they were at the time of the incident. Because these clients are usually young and healthy, this may be their first encounter with a physical condition that requires ongoing and invasive medical attention. They may be very frightened about their health, themselves, and their future, and they may be struggling to integrate traumatic medical procedures or medical emergencies. Important for both the clinician and the patient to recognize is that reproductive disorders are never merely medical conditions but, rather, carry enormous psychological weight as well. How patients cope with their medical treatment can help steer the direction of the psychological treatment, incorporating elements of cognitive behavioral therapy, psychodynamic therapy, support, bereavement, and psychoeducational interventions.

The therapist should be familiar with the various tests and procedures that are common in an infertility work-up (described in Chapter 1). A visit to a neonatal intensive care unit, for example, provides the clinician with an invaluable taste for what parents with premature babies experience. Likewise, having an understanding of the most frequent medical diagnoses for both men and women is extremely valuable. Patients feel a sense of relief if they don't have to explain to their therapist what a myomectomy is or what the symptoms of polycystic ovaries are. One patient, who had previously seen a therapist who did not specialize in the field, felt reassured by her new therapist's knowledge of reproductive issues. "Not only did I have to teach my previous therapist about IVF," she said, "but also about the emotional ups and downs I was having. I'm so glad I don't have to waste time explaining things to you." Patients resent having to educate their therapists on the various medical interventions they must endure, adding more time and expense to their already full load (Klock, 2006).

There are times when a patient's medical history is directly related to their reproductive trauma. For example, cancer patients, both male and female, are at risk of loss of reproductive function, either because of the type of cancer, the severity of the disease, the patient's age, or the treatment protocol for the particular type of cancer they have (Simon, Lee, Partridge, & Runowicz, 2005). These patients experience a double psychological blow: Naturally, survival is the primary concern, but they also must contend with trying to preserve their fertility in the process. Prior to treatment, a man may be able to bank his sperm by cryopreservation; the options for women, however, are more complex. If a woman does not have a partner, she may opt to freeze oocytes, which has had limited success for a positive pregnancy outcome (Oktay, Cil, & Bang, 2006). Alternatively, she can undergo IVF, fertilize her eggs either with her partner's sperm or with a donor's, and then freeze the resulting embryos. The problem with doing IVF is that it can take 6 to 8 weeks, and the cancer treatment may not be able to be delayed for that long. Additionally, ovarian stimulation may be contraindicated if the type of tumor is estrogen-sensitive (Simon et al., 2005). The grieving process for these patients is made that much more complex in having to cope with a life-threatening disease as well as the potential loss of fertility.

History of Previous Reproductive Events

As part of assessing medical history, special attention should be paid to the patient's history of other pregnancies and their resolution. An earlier, unplanned pregnancy may have ended in a miscarriage or an abortion, or the patient may have relinquished a child in an adoption. It is important to evaluate the effects such events might have on their current reproductive crisis. There is controversy in the literature about the impact of abortion on the mental health of women. According to the American Psychological Association (2005), the psychological risks associated with abortion are low.

Other studies, however, suggest that there may be a link between abortion and psychological problems, including depression, anxiety, substance abuse, and low self-esteem (Fergusson, Horwood, & Ridder, 2006; Reardon, Cougle, Rue, Shuping, Coleman, & Ney, 2003; Reardon & Cougle, 2002).

Whether or not a woman experienced psychological sequelae from a previous unwanted pregnancy, a new reproductive crisis can lead to many new feelings about past choices. It is important for therapists to understand that this phenomenon can happen for men as well (Haftek, 2008). The personal decisions that were made years earlier often take on a different slant and new meaning when one is faced with reproductive difficulties. As patients struggle to understand why their current problems are occurring, it can be tempting for them to rewrite history, experiencing self-blame and guilt for the previously adaptive decisions. It can be quite surprising when feelings about a previous unwanted pregnancy, which had been satisfactorily resolved and not of undue psychological consequence, suddenly give rise to feelings of confusion, sadness, and grief. When considered in the context of the reproductive story, it is easy to see how an unwanted pregnancy could change a person's script. The therapist can help by pointing out how the client's story shifted to incorporate a previous undesired pregnancy and must shift again when the now-desired child is so difficult to attain. It can help to label the earlier abortion as a reproductive trauma or loss in its own right, even if it was the right choice, and to suggest that the current trauma is stacked on the first. The irony, of course, is that for many women, as well as men, having had a previous pregnancy—solid proof of their fertility—gave them the sense that it would be quite easy to get pregnant again.

Beth, a 34-year-old woman, had two early miscarriages and has been unable to conceive at all in over a year. She spoke poignantly about her certainty that her problems were caused by an abortion she had when she was 19. "When I got pregnant, my boyfriend and I didn't tell anyone about it. We knew it wasn't right for either of us to have a baby at that time and it wasn't difficult deciding to abort. He came with me to the doctor's and stayed with me until I felt well. We gradually drifted apart, but it was all quite amicable. I rarely, if ever, thought about the abortion, and never doubted our decision—until now." Grown up and married, Beth has revisited her abortion with each painful miscarriage. "I think that for all these years, I have missed that baby," she cried. "Every time I miscarry, I lose another chance to make it up to that baby. Maybe I should have had it." Wracked with guilt and sadness about her inability to conceive, Beth has reprocessed her history, viewing it completely differently than she had at the time. Her confidence in her own judgment has given way to self-doubt and self-blame, a view of herself as weak and nonassertive. All of this has been a way for Beth to find a justified reason for her unexplained miscarriages. Even though it is inaccurate, rewriting her history gives her a hook upon which to hang all of her frustration and sadness at her current dilemmas.

History of Other Losses

Just as an earlier unwanted pregnancy can complicate the emotional reactions to a reproductive trauma, a previous nonreproductive trauma can also add to the client's current psychological distress. Experiences such as a divorce, a death in the family, or earlier serious illness can affect one's grief reaction, especially if the earlier traumas were not fully resolved. Likewise, a history of promiscuity, venereal disease, or substance abuse can increase feelings of guilt, blame, or shame (Hart, 2002). Feelings from the past often rise to the surface when a reproductive loss occurs, making it that much harder to cope with the present. If a patient has had a history of depression, anxiety, or other mental disorder, the likelihood of an intensified reaction to the current reproductive event is high. Taking note of previous losses, the therapist can help make connections with present issues, tying together the losses, and facilitating the griefwork.

Julia, 32, lost her mother suddenly and unexpectedly when she was 13. Although she grieved this catastrophic loss, she has always been plagued by regret that she never had an opportunity to say goodbye to her mother. When Julia lost her baby when she was 5 months pregnant, she felt paralyzed by grief and terrified by the intensity of her reactions; she came to sessions and could barely speak. Although the therapist suspected that Julia's current experience was in some way intensified by the loss of her mother, she did not articulate this connection right away. She knew that Julia needed to defuse her immediate sense of trauma and sadness and would have felt misunderstood had the connection to her mother been made too soon. When Julia felt calmer, however, her therapist gently wondered if she had ever felt this way before. "I feel just like I did at 13," Julia blurted. With the loss of her baby, Julia experienced a resurgence of grief over her mother's death. Once again, she was unable to say goodbye. "Oh, I miss my mom so much," she cried. "I had always imagined her being here with me when I had a baby." Not only did Julia lose her baby, but she had also looked forward to "somehow connecting with my mom again by becoming a mom—now I can't do that." By eventually understanding how her mother's death was connected to her current loss, Julia was able to separate the two experiences and grieve them individually, rendering each less overwhelming. As she became more comfortable verbalizing her feelings, Julia's therapist also encouraged her to reconnect with her mother emotionally, and in turn, with her lost baby. She suggested that Julia go visit her mother's grave, something she had not done in years. She also encouraged Julia to write a letter to her mother to tell her about her life and the loss of her baby and to say goodbye. Julia benefited not only from the understanding of her emotions but also from the concrete, guided grieving that the therapist helped her do.

History of Sexual, Emotional, or Physical Abuse

As part of getting to know the patient over time, the therapist should investigate other circumstances in a patient's life that might generate feelings of self-blame and guilt. If a patient has had a history of abuse, for example, the effects of the current reproductive trauma may be magnified. The shame and self-blame these patients experience with infertility or a pregnancy failure may reevoke similar feelings from their past (Watson, 2005). Patients who have been abused as a child—sexually, emotionally, or physically—sometimes feel as if they don't deserve to have children and see the difficulty achieving parenthood as a sign that they shouldn't. Others may feel violated by the invasive procedures of assisted reproductive technology, once again feeling objectified and helpless as they did during childhood abuse (Watson, 2005). These feelings may be even more intense when a patient is enduring the pain and fear of a miscarriage, which may be experienced as an assault. The therapist must be sensitive in exploring these issues and help make the distinction between the past and current traumas. It is important for the therapist to understand that there may be two—or more—situations that need to be grieved: the current reproductive trauma and the trauma of the past.

Assessment of Nonreproductive Cases

Our clinical experience suggests that *all* new patients should be assessed for reproductive issues, even if it is not the presenting problem. This holds true for patients of reproductive age but also for those patients who are not. Clients in their 30s may present with a variety of concerns, seemingly unrelated to reproduction. Probing their feelings, however, often reveals a preoccupation with childbearing matters, which is reasonable given the developmental concerns of this age range (Levinson, 1978, 1996). Sylvia (see Chapter 1, this volume), the young woman who had been so frightened at the stories of her mother's illness, provides a good example of this. Sylvia came for therapy because of anxiety and conflict with her partner; she had no sense of her problems being related to reproduction. In the course of therapy, however, she was able to reflect on the connection between her childhood fears and her current anxiety about becoming pregnant.

As more and more information about reproductive issues appears in the news, younger women may find themselves worried about their fertility before they have ever attempted to reproduce. Those past childbearing age may also be dealing with aspects of their story gone awry. One patient, Maria, divorced and in her early 60s, entered therapy to deal with feelings of depression since her recent retirement, but, on further reflection, a more complex view of the choices she had made in her life was revealed. Childless by choice, she wondered if she had made the right decision. With many of her friends having grandchildren, Maria felt as if she has missed out. Her fears of growing old and being alone were compounded by her friends' involvement with their children and grandchildren; she wondered what she would be able to leave behind for the future once she was gone. The introduction of this material in the therapy opened up important feelings about herself, her experiences of her own mother, and her decision, made long ago, not to have children. This example illustrates the ongoing implications of reproductive decisions over the life span. Although Maria had made what she felt was the right decision—not to have children at that stage of her life—she had not been aware of her generative needs or of the long-term unfolding of her reproductive story. It was only now, with the wisdom and maturity she had gained over time, that she appreciated the meaning of generativity and her need to find other ways to contribute to the future. Patients may enter therapy with seemingly unrelated issues, but when past reproductive events and decisions are explored, a wealth of emotional data may emerge for the therapist to work with.

On numerous occasions we have seen couples seek therapy to address relationship problems, only to find that their current troubles with each other derived from previous infertility or a pregnancy loss. Asking about their reproductive history can reveal buried feelings harbored against each other. All too often, a client may have accepted his or her partner's attitudes about having children at the beginning of a relationship, without fully exploring what it might mean in the future. George, for example, had two teenage children from a previous marriage. He had made it clear to his new wife, Gail, that he was not interested in having any more children. Even though she knew his feelings when they married, she thought she could persuade him to change his mind. Her anger and disillusionment, and her strong desire to have a child "of her own," became the root of the problems between them. At age 41, with childbearing time running out for Gail, she was furious, with a sense of loss and powerlessness in the relationship; on the other hand, George felt as if Gail broke her end of the bargain, and he was equally angry with her.

In this situation, the therapist needs to be able to express empathy for both members of the couple and to underline that neither of them is trying to hurt the other. It can be helpful to meet with each of them separately to clarify the source of their feelings. In the case just mentioned, for example, the therapist investigated George's refusal to consider having another child. Privately, he was able to acknowledge that it wasn't so much that he would never be willing to have another child as that he felt so judged and criticized by his wife as being selfish and controlling. He was so angry that he could not really have compassion for her longing for a child and the sense of loss she was experiencing. He also acknowledged that he was afraid to become a father again. He felt that the strain of parenthood had been part of the rift between him and his first wife, and he feared it would happen again in this marriage, although the conflicts over this issue were threatening the marriage already. He also worried about becoming an older father, fearing that he would not be able to keep up with young kids or fit in with young parents. He "just didn't feel that he had it in him."

Gail, on the other hand, struggled with feeling powerless and infantilized in the relationship. The daughter of a controlling mother, Gail bristled under what she felt was George's control of the decision. She also felt an imperative to have a child so that she could "do it differently" than her own mother had, to regain a sense of control over her own life and self. The therapist was kind but very direct with Gail. "It is clear that you want a child very much. That is very understandable, and not impossible. It just may not be possible with this particular husband. You are not as controlled and trapped as you feel. You can make a choice to leave the relationship to have a child with someone else. That is in your hands. But it is important to remember that your struggles over control with your husband do not derive just from his feelings about having a child—they date much farther back than your marriage." When Gail was reminded that she did have choices, she felt less trapped and then less angry at her husband. At that point, she was able to listen to his feelings and fears, without panicking that he was thwarting her plans. She was also able to see that some of her control issues needed to be worked out in therapy, not in the marriage.

This therapeutic intervention allowed Gail to think about herself and her situation differently; consequently, her attitude and behavior changed as well. After much reflection, Gail realized that her marriage was the most important part of her life and that she did not want to give it up. She and George were finally able to talk about their fears and their options and chose not to have another child. She became more accepting of her husband and more able to enjoy her role as stepmother to her husband's children.

A reproductive history is also important to gather when working with a child. When parents bring a child for treatment, it can be useful to learn from them as much as possible about that child's conception and birth, as part of obtaining the developmental history of the child. If there had been a prior reproductive trauma, for example, the subsequent child may be exhibiting behavioral problems because of the parent's unresolved grief. Similarly, if the birth had been high risk or complicated, the parent's anxiety and subsequent attachment to the child may be skewed. Far more often than therapists realize, a reproductive trauma is part of the family's history. An important intervention may be to label for the parents that they had experienced a true trauma previously. "Wow, you guys have been through a lot. And now, to be so worried about your little boy must feel overwhelming. You show remarkable fortitude to be able to focus on your son's needs when you yourselves must feel so raw inside." This comment not only highlights their anxiety but their strengths as well. Even a brief psychoeducational comment, paired with an empathic one, can do much to help parents feel understood and relieve at least some of their anxiety. Sometimes, it is useful to meet with each parent separately to ascertain their perceptions and viewpoints; it all becomes data in the effort to understand their child.

THE DIAGNOSTIC SPECTRUM

Before discussing how to treat this population, a look at some of the typical diagnoses is in order. As part of the assessment process, it is important to try to tease apart preexisting conditions from those deriving from the current problem. Because of the intensity of feelings that reproductive losses produce, many preexisting conditions, especially depression and anxiety, can be exacerbated. The patient who has a tendency toward anxiety disorders, for example, is likely to exhibit more intensified symptoms of anxiety while undergoing treatment. Furthermore, a study of women undergoing infertility treatment suggests that there is an increase in distress over time (Berg & Wilson, 1991). Additional research indicates a peak in distress and depressive symptoms between the 2nd and 3rd year of treatment (Domar, Broome, Zuttermeister, Seibel, & Friedman, 1992). Clients have described a "lack of reserves" in their ability to cope. As one patient put it, "I feel like a rubber band that has been stretched too far. I'm just not bouncing back."

Defense mechanisms that in the past might have helped a patient manage difficult emotional situations may fail to adequately bolster them through this trying time; remember, some of their defenses were relinquished the moment they decided to try to conceive. The narcissistic injury creates an overwhelming loss of self-worth; how can everyone else achieve having a baby—seemingly with such ease? The sense of self may feel fragmented and diminished; it then becomes the task of the therapist to help rebuild and reconstruct the positive sense of self (Leon, 1996). Reminding patients of their many strengths and assets, teaching them to compartmentalize their reproductive self from the rest of who they are, can help to rebuild self-esteem.

Affective Disorders

As previously mentioned, reproductive patients often exhibit symptoms of depression. There are numerous studies documenting mood changes in infertile patients (for a review, see American Society for Reproductive Medicine, 1996). Given the number of losses incurred—including the loss of identity, social standing, marital or relational satisfaction, and hope for the future—it is not surprising that patients would have depressive reactions. It can be helpful to think of depression as a normal and to-be-expected response to this life-altering event. As discussed in Chapter 3, reflecting on the multiple losses that occur from a biopsychosocial viewpoint, it makes sense that failed attempts at pregnancy would contribute to depressive reactions: The body isn't working as it is supposed to, the opportunities for psychological growth are hampered, and the social alienation from peers who are having children is powerful (Gerrity, 2001). Grief reactions are common, whether the couple experienced the loss of a real baby or a fantasized one. It is not surprising that patients exhibit overwhelming feelings of sadness, despair, weepiness, and irritability. Avoidance and isolation tend to be natural consequences of reproductive trauma. Patients feel the need to protect themselves from the outside world, and yet this may play a part in heightening their depressed mood.

Angry responses often take the individual or couple by surprise and may challenge core beliefs about themselves and about each other. Couples who find themselves uncharacteristically argumentative may not readily attribute their irritability to their loss. Not only are they angry with each other, they may also be angry with their doctors, their family, and friends. They may turn their anger inward and blame themselves, thus contributing to their depressed mood. They may question long-held religious beliefs: Their anger may be addressed to a god they no longer trust. Although there are numerous differences in the ways women and men respond to and cope with this crisis (discussed in Chapter 5), women more stereotypically exhibit tears, vulnerability, and lethargy. Men, on the other hand, may feel helpless and frustrated in not being able to solve the problem. They may also try to escape their feelings by working more, indulging in greater substance abuse, or avoiding their emotions by spending more time in other distracting activities. The clinician can be a sounding board as the couple airs their differences. Pointing out that it is normal for each partner to manage the loss in his or her own way—neither is "right or wrong," just different—can bring relief to otherwise seemingly insurmountable tensions.

Anxiety Disorders

Anxiety reactions are also prevalent; the loss of control over one's reproductive life intensifies distress. There is a tendency to believe that if things went wrong before, they will again. When one experiences a pregnancy loss, for example, it is difficult to believe that a subsequent pregnancy will result in a live birth, even though the odds are favorable that all will proceed as it should. It is an understatement to say that these patients and their relationships are stressed. Likewise, the chronic nature of infertility, month after month of anticipation and defeat, wears away at even the most robust relationship. Both men and women report lower satisfaction in their marriage and sexual life with their partner when dealing with infertility (Slade, Emery, & Lieberman, 1997; Verhaak, Smeenk, van Minnen, Kremer, & Kraaimaat, 2005). The level of distress in infertile women has been compared with that in cancer patients, women with heart disease, and those with HIV+ status (Domar, Zuttermeister, & Friedman, 1993).

Some of the anxiety that clients experience may present itself in an obsessive-like manner. Infertility patients are often preoccupied with their efforts to have a baby, spending years and enormous sums of money to achieve their goal. Often, we have heard a disgruntled spouse complaining of the endless hours his partner spends researching the Internet for the latest medical innovation. It is true that the medical options offer a feeling of unending hope, making it more difficult for infertile clients to end treatment and consider alternate family-building choices. The idea of trying one more time, in spite of poor odds, is emotionally gripping; everyone has heard of someone who, on her eighth IVF cycle, finally became pregnant. With the carrot of a potential baby dangling in front of their nose, it's no wonder clients become fixated and trapped in the process.

It's important to note another aspect of endless rounds of treatment: Some infertility patients get caught in the cycle of repeated attempts in order to forestall admitting defeat. The desire for a baby may keep patients stuck in this chapter of their life, if they are unwilling to consider other options—even to simply take a break (if medically okayed). If an individual or couple persist in trying, they can avoid the full extent of their grief, steer clear of facing the enormous sense of failure, and evade tackling other family-building options. It is especially difficult if their medical team suggests that a tweak of medication or a change in timing will do the trick. The concept of the reproductive story can be helpful at this juncture in reminding patients that this is just a chapter—albeit a very important one—in the opus of their life. By placing this crisis into the larger context of their life, the therapist can help clients keep it in perspective.

Symptoms of posttraumatic stress disorder (PTSD) are yet another anxiety reaction to reproductive loss. As previously mentioned, patients can experience flashbacks, dissociation, numbness, and avoidance of places or things that may trigger a negative reaction. One patient found it impossible to drive past the hospital where she learned of the demise of her pregnancy. Another couldn't face returning to her previous reproductive endocrinologist after a failed IVF cycle. Seeing the staff, who had been so hopeful and encouraging to her partner and her, proved to be unbearable. She felt as if she had somehow let them down and decided to continue treatment at another clinic instead.

Even mundane, day-to-day chores may elicit PTSD-like reactions. Seeing a pregnant woman picking up dry cleaning, for instance, may set into motion a chain of emotional reactions that feel excruciating. The point is that patients' defenses are fragile. Seemingly innocuous situations can generate a whole host of reactions that, under normal circumstances, would not appear. By working with clients to build a "suit of armor" to manage the daily strains they face, the therapist, in essence, is helping them to bolster existing defenses and/or create new ones.

SUMMARY

As this chapter illustrates, reproductive patients enter therapy at all different phases, for many different problems. Sometimes, they don't even realize that the crux of their difficulties is related to reproductive issues until explored in therapy. Therefore, with every new client, it is helpful to include probes for their reproductive histories as part of the initial assessment.

When patients come in specifically for reproductive issues, the initial focus should be on the immediate trauma and loss, dealing as one would in a crisis intervention. Over time, a more in-depth history will naturally unfold as the therapist listens for, looks for, and asks about a number of themes. These include:

- inviting the patient to tell the story of his or her reproductive trauma and loss;
- asking about details of his or her experience, including specific medical information;
- asking about how his or her partner has handled the crisis;
- taking note of symptoms of depression, anxiety, PTSD, and obsessive–compulsive disorder;
- listening for where the developmental tasks of adulthood have gone awry;
- reviewing history of previous trauma and loss, whether reproductive or not; and
- assessing the different coping styles of each partner and how they might create conflict.

As treatment unfolds, the therapist will know more precisely the needs of each patient. Sometimes, he or she needs support and validation of feelings; at other times, psychoeducation about the reproductive story, about the kinds of emotions that are expected and normal, about the grief process, and about the conflict it can create within the relationship all can be very useful and provide a great deal of relief. If over time it becomes evident that the current trauma is complicated by prior losses, other conflicts within the relationship, or unresolved issues relating to family of origin, then deeper, more dynamically oriented psychotherapy can prove to be of utmost value.

It is imperative that the therapist remain flexible and neutral when working with reproductive patients. She or he must be open to working in a crisis-intervention mode initially and be patient in allowing the additional needs and meaning of the reproductive events to emerge. Often, validating and normalizing the fact that these events truly are a crisis is a crucial first step in helping the patient to feel understood and to gain some relief.

5

GRIEVING A REPRODUCTIVE LOSS

How does one grieve a pregnancy loss? Or a baby that never was? How does one fully grieve when in the midst of trying to conceive? How do couples manage their feelings while mourning a death when there should have been life? Although the loss of an adult loved one is painful and sad, the loss of a longed for pregnancy is unique and needs to be recognized as such by clinicians.

Because there is a fundamental biological imperative to protect and nurture one's offspring, when a baby dies before or at birth, parents feel as if they have failed in the most basic way. The loss hits home on a primal level. Quite literally, because of the biological and physical connection between a mother and child-in-utero, a mother may experience the loss as if a part of herself has died. Parents have not only lost a baby, but they have lost their hopes and dreams for that child (Rando, 1985, 1986). As Arnold and Gemma described it, "the loss of an adult is the loss of the past; the loss of a baby is the loss of the future" (Arnold & Gemma, 1994, as cited in Robinson, Baker, & Nackerud, 1999). The future—which should have been filled with caring for a baby—is now held in dread. These losses shake the very foundation of trust in a coherent, safe, and predictable world.

Often, individuals or couples feel alone in their grief; they may feel alienated from others who they believe cannot understand. Indeed, they may not understand it themselves and struggle to find meaning in their inability to conceive or in the death of their baby. Although parents who have had a stillbirth or neonatal loss may utilize the customs of their religion and hospital support to help with the grief process (although the latter is a fairly recent phenomenon), there are virtually no rituals or cultural norms for grieving a miscarriage or infertility. And yet each month when a woman gets her period, each cycle that fails to result in a pregnancy, is a kind of "mini-death" and needs to be grieved just as if someone in the family had died; indeed, a member of the family *has* died.

While Chapter 4 focused on initial assessment, this chapter addresses the complicated task of grieving infertility and pregnancy loss, a huge component of the psychotherapy. It discusses various models of bereavement and how they apply specifically to this population. Differences in the ways that individuals grieve are illustrated with case examples. Therapeutic interventions, such as the creation of grief rituals to help fully acknowledge these losses, are suggested. Recognizing and mourning the multiple losses associated with infertility and pregnancy loss is crucial for clients; it allows them to repair the damage to their sense of self and to make decisions about future family planning.

MODELS OF BEREAVEMENT

Theories of grief and mourning in Western culture have evolved since Freud, in 1917, first proposed the need to hypercathect and then decathect the image of the deceased (Rothaupt & Becker, 2007). According to this model, following an initial period of emotional discharge and acknowledgment of the death, the mourners must sever the bonds with the deceased to build new relationships. The ultimate goal of grieving was to free oneself from the emotional attachments to the deceased. Lindemann (1944), expanding on Freud's ideas, discussed the idea of *griefwork*, which entails acknowledgment of the person's absence, feeling the loss, and adjusting to life without the loved one in order to form new relationships. Lindemann (1944) also noted that grief can be delayed or can reemerge long after the death occurred and may be dependent on the attachment and relationship to the deceased.

Other models of bereavement—the stage theories—are based on the notion that grief follows a particular progression and that one stage must be completed before moving on to the next. Kubler-Ross (1969), in her seminal work with terminally ill patients, developed a five-stage theory: denial (this can't be happening to me), anger (why is this happening?), bargaining (if I promise to do better, then this will not happen), despair or resignation (a loss of hope: there is no way to stop this from happening), and finally acceptance (it has happened). One of the drawbacks to the stage theory model of bereavement is that people do not necessarily grieve in a set order or totally complete a stage before entering the next. It is important for the clinician to remember that it is not uncommon for people, especially reproductive patients, to experience all of these stages in a short amount of time and then return to prior stages. If the stages are taken too literally, it may make the bereaved feel as if they are doing something wrong and not grieving "correctly," which further diminishes their self-esteem. This can be especially difficult for couples, when one partner is at a different stage from the other, or thinks the other "should be over it."

The question of whether one can truly detach from the deceased has led to more recent theories, which in fact more adequately match the clinical experience of parental bereavement. Based on John Bowlby's (1969) attachment theory, the idea of a continued emotional bond between the bereaved and the deceased has emerged. Prior to this wave of research, the task for the bereaved was to disengage emotionally from the deceased. In fact, for much of the 20th century, it was considered a sign of pathological grieving if a person had continued bonds with the deceased (Klass, 2006). However, researchers have shown that mourners do have a continued sense of connection with the deceased—by having positive memories, feeling their presence, talking about (or to) them in their mind, or saving meaningful belongings—and that this can bring comfort to the bereaved. Rather than breaking bonds, a new and transformed relationship with the deceased can emerge, one in which the survivors learn to live without the person and to find comfort in the memories (Capitulo, 2005).

CONTINUED BONDS, ATTACHMENT THEORY, AND THE REPRODUCTIVE STORY

Prior to 1970, grief following a miscarriage or stillbirth was not readily acknowledged. In fact, these losses were treated as nonevents; families were routinely told to simply get on with their lives and not dwell on it (Brownlee & Oikonen, 2004). Although this advice, offered by family and friends, as well as by the medical community, was well meaning, the bereaved parents were left feeling confused and unsupported; to grieve "properly," they had to disregard their emotions: an impossible task. It was taboo to discuss these losses: One woman, in her mid-70s, was heartened to learn about a support group for couples who had a perinatal loss. "There was nothing like that when I had my miscarriage," she said. "Nobody talked about it; it just got shoved under the carpet. But it's not something that goes away. I still feel upset whenever I think about it." This, after over 50 years had past.

Rather than thinking of these losses as nonevents, therapists have more recently come to view them as potentially devastating for the bereaved individual or couple. There is now more recognition that attachment exists between parent and child long before the infant's birth. Indeed, as we have been emphasizing throughout, it is our assertion that the parent–child bond, that is, the reproductive story, begins far earlier, prior to conception, prior to a committed relationship (Jaffe, Diamond, & Diamond, 2005). The seeds of attachment that parents have for their child-to-be most likely starts with the tie they have with their own parents and the desire to emulate them. In essence, it begins with the early reproductive stories—the ideas and fantasies of what it will be like to have a child and be a parent. As discussed in Chapter 1, the reproductive story makes up a large part of one's identity. With infertility, or when a pregnancy fails, the loss is not only perceived as a loss of connection with the hoped-for child but also as a personal failure, the loss of part of the self.

With this model, it becomes clear that the attachment to the child and to the idea of becoming a parent, that is, the nature of the reproductive story and parental identity, are critical factors in understanding the extent of the loss for each individual. Although there are periods in which attachment is heightened—feeling fetal movement, giving birth, and caring for the baby—the bond begins much earlier and includes thinking about and planning the pregnancy (Peppers & Knapp, 1980). By the time the child is born, mothers have a sense of knowing the child, with expectations of how the infant will fit into the life of the family (Robinson et al, 1999; Rubin, 1975).

Rather than detaching from the deceased, as early bereavement theory suggested, the continuing bonds literature supports the idea that, although the physical relationship with the deceased ends, a new relationship, based on memories, can be a part of successful mourning (Rothaupt & Becker, 2007). But how does one form a relationship based on memories when—as with infertility or pregnancy loss—there are none, or only painful ones? The reproductive story can play a vital part here: The therapist's exploration of the hopes and dreams of would-be parents allows them to maintain a sense of attachment with their longed-for child by incorporating it into their story, which can help reestablish their sense of self.

It is important for clinicians to understand that the intensity or length of grief after a reproductive loss is not determined by the duration of the pregnancy. Reactions can be affected by many variables: Whether the pregnancy was desired or not, if there had been previous perinatal or other losses, the difficulty and length of time it took to conceive, the amount of outside intervention necessary for conception (i.e., in vitro fertilization [IVF]), whether there are any living children, the nature of the parents' relationship, and the woman's age (Bennett, Litz, Lee, & Maguen, 2005; Conway & Valentine, 1987; Lasker & Toedter, 2000). A woman who has suffered an early miscarriage, for example, may experience some of the same feelings as a woman who has had a third-trimester perinatal loss. Even though the child—whether in utero or a neonate—may not have been with the parent for very long, there is a bond that forms, and the loss is by no means less significant (Robinson, et al., 1999). Attachment may have increased for the woman with the third-trimester loss because of fetal movement (Peppers & Knapp, 1980), but the grief reaction may be just as intense; in both cases, her baby has died.

In a similar vein, two women suffering a perinatal loss at the same gestational point may have diverse reactions to the loss. A pregnant teen with ambivalence toward motherhood may have a very different response to a miscarriage than a 38-year-old woman who has had several years of infertility. Although both have a reproductive story, it is fair to assume that their focus is completely different. Both have had reproductive stories that have gone awry: We can presume that the teen did not plan on becoming pregnant, may have had thoughts of having children "someday," and may be relieved that she miscarried, whereas the 38-year-old with a history of infertility is likely to be devastated by the event. Their responses have less to do with the point of time in their pregnancies that the loss occurred than with the point of time in their lives. In assessing patients, the clinician must factor in the meaning of the pregnancy, their readiness and wish to take on the responsibility of becoming a parent, and the extent and intensity of the attachment. "Accurate assessment of the degree of attachment is a critical factor" (Robinson et. al., 1999, p. 265).

With advances in ultrasound technology, people have an opportunity to bond visually with their baby long before past generations would even have known they were pregnant; this serves to increase attachment earlier in the pregnancy. In a study of men's reactions to their partner's miscarriage, Puddifoot and Johnson (1999) found that men who had seen ultrasound images of their baby had a significantly stronger grief reaction to the miscarriage than those men who did not. Infertility patients going through in vitro fertilization can see their embryo in a Petri dish prior to implantation. One patient proudly displayed a photograph of her embryo as part of her baby album. But even if infertility patients have no concrete, physical connection to a child, they may grieve just as intensely after each failed cycle. Greenfeld, Diamond, and DeCherney (1988) described the symptoms of grief after a failed IVF as mirroring those of women suffering a pregnancy loss, and they suggested that a woman's response could be predicted by her attachment to the anticipated pregnancy. Although an infertility patient may not have achieved a pregnancy during the course of treatment, the attachment to the idealized child may produce an intense grief reaction to the failure equal to that of a pregnancy loss.

Regardless of the type of loss, it is important for the clinician to assess and understand what the meaning of the pregnancy, or the hoped for pregnancy, is for the individual or couple. The expectations about parenthood and the hoped-for child contribute to an increased sense of failure and loss (Robinson et al., 1999). As discussed in the following sections, recognizing the attachment that begins in preconception, the mental health practitioner can help families through the grief process through validation of emotions, development of rituals, and the use of the reproductive story as a means of continuing the relationship with the lost baby.

GRIEVING PERINATAL LOSS AND INFERTILITY

As painful as it is when a loved one has died, grieving that loss is made easier by the structure of culture and religion. The rituals surrounding death vary from culture to culture, but most involve family and friends coming together to remember and honor the deceased. Eulogies at funerals, for example, celebrate the person's life by recognizing and sharing treasured memories. Reminiscing about the person—recalling the good times and the bad—is a natural phenomenon that aids and enhances the mourning process. But with a perinatal loss or infertility, the memories—what few there are—tend to be negative; they may consist of hospital procedures, medical emergencies, or maybe just the crushing disappointment of a negative pregnancy test.

As discussed previously, neither feelings of attachment nor the experience of loss are dependent on the duration of the pregnancy. In the grieving process, however, the length of time a pregnancy lasts can make a difference, in terms of whether there are accepted cultural rituals and support from family and friends. To date, there are a number of socially sanctioned practices following a death after a premature birth, stillbirth, or other neonatal demise but not for loss from a miscarriage or infertility. For example, it is now common practice after a stillbirth or neonatal death in a hospital for the staff to persuade parents to see and hold their baby. Parents may at first reject this idea, but later, as they reflect on that moment, they are very appreciative of the time they were able to spend with their infant. Women who are unable to hold their baby because of medical complications describe feeling robbed of their only chance to connect with their child. Seeing their child is also a relief to many parents; the fantasies of what he or she looks like are often much worse than the reality. It has been reported, for example, that mothers who did not see their deceased baby dreamt their child was a monster (Kroth, Garcia, Hallgren, LeGrue, Ross, & Scalise, 2004). Parents are also encouraged to name their child, unless it is not a cultural norm to do so. Holding and/or naming the baby helps make the child and the experience real, which facilitates the grief process. Likewise, having photographs of the deceased infant and preparing a memory box are concrete ways of remembering the baby. Along with photographs, the box may include locks of the baby's hair, handprints and footprints, hand or foot casts, or a hospital name bracelet. Some parents take comfort in writing letters to their baby or they may include a meaningful poem in the box expressing their heartfelt feelings. These tangible remembrances provide some solace for the bereaved parents.

Additionally, many people choose to have a funeral or memorial service for their baby. Not only is this a validation of the loss, but these rituals themselves, religious or not, also serve as important memories for the surviving family. Many families choose to visit the grave site of the deceased baby on a regular basis, bringing flowers, gifts, or even food. One family asked friends and relatives to meet at a beach and write a personal note to their baby; they then placed her ashes in a canister with the messages, and "sent her spirit out to sea." Another family had a private ceremony: On a balloon, each parent attached his or her own letter to the baby and sent it off. (The parents continue to do so every year on the date their son died.) Yet another woman chose to plant a flowering bush that blooms each year during the anniversary of her baby's death.

These rituals and symbolic remembrances are in keeping with the continuing bonds theory of bereavement. Rather than withdrawing emotional energy from the deceased, a connection continues and gets woven into the fabric of the family's life (Cote-Arsenault, 2003). The mental health professional can help parents by validating the need for this link with their baby, suggesting meaningful rituals, and eliciting concrete ways to ensure that their child will not be forgotten.

For someone who has had a miscarriage or for those who are struggling with infertility, however, mourning is more complicated, given the absence of socially validated grieving rituals. These losses, although not less meaningful, are less tangible, less recognized by society at large, and have no prescribed ceremonies to guide parents through bereavement. As devastating as a stillbirth or neonatal death is to parents, the mourning process is facilitated by the reality of the baby's body (McGreal, Evans, & Burrows, 1997). When there is no actual body to grieve over, as in a miscarriage, an ectopic pregnancy, or with infertility, grief may feel illegitimate. Doka (1989) defined this phenomenon as *disenfranchised grief*, which refers to grief that is not publicly recognized or acknowledged and therefore is minimized by society at large. If a relationship does not meet the unwritten rules of a sanctioned loss, then the survivors may feel deprived of their grief. Many relationships fall into this category, such as the loss of a former spouse, the loss of a gay or lesbian partner, or the loss a birth parent experiences when relinquishing a child. Parents who experience infertility and/or miscarriage are prime risks for disenfranchised grief. There are no rules for the way these losses should be mourned, no models to follow for the bereaved or for their close relations. The well-meaning things people say—"You can have another" or "It's for the best" or "Just relax"—totally miss the mark, leaving the bereaved feeling alone with their loss and completely misunderstood. Indeed, often, couples literally are alone with their feelings, as the only people who may be aware that a significant loss has occurred may be the couple themselves and perhaps their doctor. As one patient remarked, "If I told my boss that I needed to attend my aunt's funeral, the time would readily be granted. But if I told him that I was grieving because I got my period again this month, he would think I was nuts."

Even with accepted rituals and memorials, parents may feel disenfranchised in their grief, especially after some time has passed since the loss, and they are expected to be over it. Many report feeling support when the loss first occurs, but as time goes on, fewer people acknowledge their grief or want to discuss it. Celeste, for example, had been devastated when she lost her baby at 24 weeks gestation. She immediately began therapy and attended a support group to help her grieve. She was even prepared for what she had learned were "anniversary reactions," when she felt a resurgence of sadness a year after her loss.

Celeste was less prepared for her depression another year later, 2 years after her trauma. Pregnant again, and in her 8th month, she had actually lost track of the date of her previous loss; she had relaxed once this pregnancy had passed the 24-week mark and was excitedly preparing for the birth. She was, therefore, shocked one day to find herself slipping into a deep depression, and she had no idea why this was happening. Reluctant to "spoil" this last part of her pregnancy, she called her previous therapist. It was startling to her when her therapist reminded her of the time of year and pointed out that it was the anniversary of her loss. It was very helpful for Celeste to realize that anniversary reactions can occur years after the initial trauma; it was important not only to be aware of the date but even to plan for it. Her therapist encouraged her to write a note to her lost baby, expressing both her love and sadness but also sharing the news that a new baby was coming. She felt comforted by being able to reassure her lost baby that the new child would never replace it, that it would always have a place in her heart. Unburdening herself and marking the anniversary in this way allowed Celeste to move past her grief and regain her sense of joy at the upcoming birth.

Clinicians need to be aware that sometimes, after a perinatal loss, bereaved parents can become developmentally impeded by their grief. In an attempt to maintain bonds with their baby, for example, they may try to hold time at a standstill and avoid making decisions or changes in their lives. They may feel guilty for moving forward, as if by doing so they would be dishonoring or abandoning their deceased child. One woman, who had lost her son when he was delivered prematurely, had begun feeling better, until her husband received a promotion. His new position required them to move to another city, which meant leaving the apartment where she had been pregnant. The upcoming move triggered enormous anxiety and a sense of loss all over again; the memories of her son were tied to that space, and moving, to her, meant leaving her baby behind. While empathizing with her sadness, the therapist helped the patient brainstorm about how she could maintain her connection to her baby, even if she was physically distant from him. The patient realized that if she took photographs of his gravesite and of the apartment where he would have lived, she could imbue these with meaning, create a tangible representation of her baby, allowing her to take him—and her memories of him—with her. The therapist also commented that, although the patient would be away from him, she still always knew where he was, and she could visit him in her mind and memories; she even noted that if the patient wished, she could travel to physically visit the grave site if she needed to. Although the patient did not anticipate doing this, being given "permission" to consider it made her feel less like her connection to her baby was being severed by the move. Through these ideas and plans, the patient was able to realize that, although she could not have her son, she never needed to be distant from her love and memories of him.

WHEN COUPLES GRIEVE DIFFERENTLY

Just as an individual may experience loss differently, depending on its meaning, couples may also grieve differently. This may be due to differences in cognitive style or to emotional issues that are specific to one member of the couple. It is normal that people grieve at different times and in different ways, but this can create tension and misunderstanding within the relationship, especially in the context of disenfranchised grief that has no obvious method to follow. Feelings of impatience and resentment may emerge when one member of the couple struggles with his or her feelings more than the other or expresses them in a way the other just doesn't understand. When one person is needier or more depressed, he or she may not be able to move forward as readily as the partner, complicating the process of deciding what steps to take next.

This was problematic for Kelly and Liz, a lesbian couple, following the miscarriage of a baby conceived using an anonymous sperm donor. Because Kelly was older, it had been an easy decision that Liz would be the partner to carry the baby; they were both shocked and heartbroken when Liz miscarried at 18 weeks. Although they were both devastated and mutually supportive after the miscarriage, Kelly seemed to "bounce back" more easily than Liz. She went back to work, was eager to socialize, and was already looking forward to trying again. Liz, however, remained grief stricken. She could not imagine going back to work, and she avoided going out, because she did not want to have to deal with people's reactions. Liz's grief was intensified by the fact that she had been carrying the baby, had loved being pregnant, and had just begun to feel the baby move. She also acknowledged feeling guilty that she had been the one to get pregnant instead of Kelly but then had been unable to "do her job." She worried that Kelly would blame her for the miscarriage, or even leave her, although when she told this to her partner, Kelly readily assured her that this was not the case.

When a couple shares a reproductive loss or the experience of infertility, they may assume that their own reaction to the loss will be the same as their partner's. But it is interesting that, often, partners will literally "take turns" processing their grief; in the matter of a short time, the tables can completely turn as the feelings of each partner switch. After 6 months or so, Liz was feeling better and was eager to try again. At that point, however, Kelly became very anxious and unsure that they should attempt another pregnancy. It emerged that Kelly had found Liz's sadness and depression very upsetting and had made efforts to counter it by diving back into her life after the loss. When Liz began to feel better, Kelly's own sadness and worry had a chance to surface. In a series of individual sessions with the therapist, Kelly also acknowledged her anger at Liz; "With Liz so upset, there was no room for my own feelings." In exploring this, Kelly realized that she had never really addressed her own sense of loss of being unable to bear a child. She had focused all of her energy on the baby that Liz was carrying. Only when Kelly had had an opportunity to process this part of her grief was the couple able to return to the decision-making process about what step to take next in their efforts to have a family.

It should also be noted that this "flip flop" between partners happens often in relationships when there is a decision to be made. The couple essentially splits the ambivalence, with one person taking one point of view ("Let's get going") and the other taking the opposite ("I am not ready"). If one person changes his or her position, the partner may also change, as if to keep a balance between them, like a seesaw. It can take time and continued negotiating for each person to come to the middle and make a shared decision.

The point to be stressed is that misunderstandings of the grief process can cause strife within the relationship and can leave one feeling as if he or she is not grieving "right." It is, indeed, rarely the case that a couple will grieve in the same way and at the same time. It is likely that they will not only have contrasting styles of grief but will also probably deal with different issues at different points in the process (Gilbert, 1996), as Kelly and Liz illustrated. On an intellectual level, they may understand and accept that these differences exist, yet, emotionally, misunderstandings and misinterpretations of the other's behavior are more common than not.

There can also be gender differences in the way that couples grieve. On the surface, it appears that men and women express grief in stereotypically different ways. The commonly held idea of how grief is conveyed—through tears, sadness, and depressed mood—is considered a feminine model. Characteristics of the feminine style of bereavement include emotional expression of the loss and a need to talk about and "process" it (Rando, 1985, 1986). Men, on the other hand, bear the stereotype of not showing their emotions; typecast in the role of the stoic partner, they typically deal with their reactions to the loss through thought, not feelings. They are less likely to talk about it (DeFrain, 1991), avoid emotional displays, and use cognitive, problem-solving strategies to cope with the loss (Rando, 1985, 1986).

Stroebe and Schut (1999) recognized the gender-related differences in grieving and proposed a dual-process model to understand how people cope with bereavement. Each person has varying degrees of both loss-orientation and restoration-orientation styles of coping. *Loss-orientation* refers to the more traditional notion of grief, with concentration and rumination on the loss and trauma, whereas *restoration-orientation* coping focuses on the things that need to be dealt with when a loss occurs, in order to rebuild one's life without the loved one (Stroebe & Schut, 1999). For successful coping with a loss, there needs to be a balance between expression of feelings and contemplation of the past and accepting the reality of the changes in one's life because of the loss. This is another type of seesawing that partners do when grieving reproductive loss. They must not only balance each other, they must also balance the grief over their loss while simultaneously looking forward, with hope, to their next procedure, their next pregnancy. At the same time one is grieving the loss, one needs to rewrite the reproductive story to restore meaning and hope for the future.

Studies have demonstrated that there are differences in how men and women grieve, but not necessarily in stereotypical ways. In comparisons of men and women following a pregnancy loss, scores on the Perinatal Grief Scale (PGS; Toedter, Lasker, & Alhadeff, 1988) indicate that although women's grief is more intense immediately following the loss ("active grief"), men have delayed effects as measured by the Difficulty in Coping and the Despair subscales of the PGS (Puddifoot & Johnson, 1999; Stinson, Lasker, Lohmann, & Toedter, 1992). Indeed, the Despair subscale is by far the most serious; it reflects an internalized response to the grief and has implications of long-term emotional effects (Toedter, et al., 1988). Men may return to work, restore a sense of control, and may seemingly get back to normal more quickly than women, but by no means does this imply that they do not have intense grief reactions.

Clinical observations suggest that, at least on the surface, men and women cope with these losses in different ways. Typically, female patients have a strong need for emotional catharsis: They cry and need to talk and express their feelings. They often feel exhausted and overwhelmed, have difficulty concentrating, want to isolate and avoid social situations, and feel anxious and/or depressed. Male patients are culturally expected—and expect themselves—to be strong and to protect and support their wives. As such, men usually assume the job, especially following pregnancy demise, of informing the family of the event and making the funeral arrangements. Similarly, when an infertility procedure is unsuccessful, a man is likely to take on the "coach–cheerleader" role, providing suggestions for future solutions as a way of comforting his partner. Although it may appear that men are functioning well, more than likely they are masking their devastation. Clinicians should be aware that men are just as likely to be suffering and should not ignore them in therapy.

One man, for example, confessed that he would cry alone in his car. He was afraid that if he cried in front of his wife, or even talked about their infertility, that she would get more upset. The irony of the situation was that she had been upset because he *hadn't* been talking about it; she didn't think he cared and was no longer sure he even wanted children. Another woman, who had experienced a stillbirth, also felt that she no longer knew her husband to be the man she had married. After returning from the hospital, she retired to the bedroom, shut the blinds, and attempted to blot out the world, when she heard some loud banging coming from another part of their house. Her husband had decided to begin renovating the kitchen. Although they had discussed plans for it before, at that particular moment it was the furthest thing from her mind; she was furious and felt he was being completely insensitive to her needs. The therapist explored the reasons for his actions: At first he had no clue what had compelled him to take on the project at that moment. His rage over their loss was clear to the therapist; she gently pointed out that his anger was so overwhelming that he needed to take some physical action. He was able to express his fury by ripping doors off cabinets and smashing countertops. Additionally, building something new was a way to overcome his feelings of helplessness; he could create something he had control over. Finally, throwing himself into this project was his way of shutting out the world and being alone with his grief. Discussing this in therapy, he was able to recognize how disconcerting his actions were to his wife. Because both were able to see that this was his way of coping with grief, they were able to open communications and gain an understanding of each other's needs. What is important for the clinician to remember is that there are many ways to cope with grief; there is no right or wrong way to mourn these losses. In fact, what might appear to be bizarre behavior, such as tearing out a kitchen, may, in fact, be a constructive coping strategy.

It is also important for the mental health practitioner not to make gender assumptions. Many women express their grief in the "masculine" style and vice versa. Martin and Doka (2000) recommended thinking of grief outside of the typical gender stereotypes. They offered two styles of grieving that are related to gender, but not necessarily determined by it: *intuitive* and *instrumental*. The intuitive griever is characterized by his or her expression of feelings; outward displays of crying and lamenting reflect what he or she is experiencing internally. He or she may have difficulty concentrating, feel disorganized and confused, and feel physically exhausted as a result. In contrast, the instrumental griever displays less intense feelings, with thinking being the dominant characteristic. Most important for the instrumental griever is the ability to master the situation. Rather than talk about feelings, these grievers rely on problem-solving strategies to regain a sense of control. Many grievers demonstrate patterns of both intuitive and instrumental styles. This "blended" pattern transcends gender, and the continuum from intuitive to instrumental may vary per individual, depending on the particular loss (Martin & Doka, 2000).

CASE EXAMPLE: ANNA AND GABRIEL

A poignant example of how disparate a couple's grief reaction can be is illustrated by Gabriel and his wife, Anna, whose son was born too early at 6 months gestation. After spending 2 months in the neonatal intensive care unit, a time filled with so much anxiety that it all felt like a nightmarish blur, their son developed a respiratory infection and died. Anna and Gabriel came in for therapy to deal with their loss and because they felt disengaged and distant from each other.

As she began therapy, Anna described feeling numb and could not come to terms with the fact that her baby was no longer with her. She seemed almost paralyzed with the sense of loss, both of the baby and of her pregnancy. Gabriel was experiencing the death of his son quite differently. He felt a deep connection to his baby, felt peace when visiting the grave site (which he did weekly), and truly felt that his son was part of his life. He talked openly about the loss with work colleagues, whom he experienced as kind and compassionate. He was very supportive of his wife but troubled at what he perceived was her disconnection from their child and, in turn, from him. Unlike Gabriel, Anna did not want to talk about the baby or visit the grave. She seemed to her husband to have shut down all of her emotions about their son, which not only worried him but also made it difficult for him to share the grieving experience with her. Gabriel felt that she pushed him away and retreated into her own sense of loss, rather than experiencing it as "their" shared loss.

In therapy, Anna revealed that her own workplace had made no acknowledgement of her baby's death. She felt alone and alienated from everyone, including her husband, who, because he seemed to feel so much better so soon, she worried could not comprehend the depth of her agony; she was bereft not only of the baby but also of the pregnancy. Although she was glad that Gabriel felt a sense of peace about their son, it also left her feeling that there was a gap between them, that they were on separate planets in their grief; in her view, he had lost a son, but she had literally lost a part of herself. It became clear to the therapist that Gabriel's was more of a restoration-orientation or instrumental grief, as he tried to return their life to some kind of normal, whereas Anna was focused on the mourning with a loss-orientation. Anna acknowledged that she shut down, feeling that it was the only way not to be overwhelmed by her pain. It was as if she was trying to pace herself, to "titrate" her sadness, and was processing the loss at a different pace from her husband.

As Anna talked about her feelings over several months, she gradually felt better, and her depression lifted. As she became more able to tolerate and verbalize her feelings, she was able to regain a sense of connection to her son. In these sessions, the therapist reassured Anna that there was not a right or wrong way to grieve and that her decision not to visit the grave did not reflect on her love for her baby. This brought Anna much relief, knowing that she could continue loving her son even in his absence and be comforted by her feelings for him.

As Anna began to feel like herself again, the therapist expected that the couple would end their therapy shortly. But one day they came in and, quite out of the blue, Gabriel, who previously had been very open and articulate, was unwilling or unable to talk. His wife commented that he had become withdrawn and irritable at home but would not tell her what was troubling him; she felt angry at his lack of communication and worried that he somehow blamed her for something. The therapist, who had felt she had a strong alliance with both Anna and Gabriel, tried to engage him to learn what was on his mind. All he could say was that he didn't know and couldn't speak. The silence continued for several sessions, and the therapist became aware that she had begun to feel the same frustration with Gabriel that his wife did. She expressed to him her puzzlement that he had shut her out and, like his wife, wondered out loud if she had done or said something to upset him. Gabriel insisted that the problem was not with either his wife or the therapist.

Stymied, the therapist stopped trying to get Gabriel to tell them what was wrong; instead, she simply asked him to describe his physical sensations. Gabriel picked up on this approach and began to talk about how he felt paralyzed, immoveable, like nothing existed and nothing mattered. He went so far as to say that he felt like he was dead inside. As he talked, he began to cry (something he had never done in session) and acknowledged how much he missed his son; having previously felt so connected to his son, Gabriel now acknowledged that only by feeling "dead" himself could he feel a bond with his baby. Although the loving attachment he had felt to his son was genuine, he had become aware that he had not fully accepted that, in fact, his baby was gone forever. Although the therapist made no comments on the shift in their roles, she was aware of the change: He had shifted to more of a loss-orientation or intuitive form of grieving while his wife moved toward a restoration-orientation. As noted previously (in the case of Kelly and Liz), this kind of role reversal is not an uncommon occurrence as couples make their way through the grieving process.

Most significantly, Gabriel was finally able to tell the therapist and his wife that he had been silent because he felt a desperate need simply to *feel* his emotions, to truly *experience* them. For him, the cognitive act of verbalizing his feelings did not relieve him but instead truncated his experience, cut off the raw emotion that he desperately needed to feel. Throughout this session, both the therapist and his wife remained quiet and simply sat with him. Without words, he felt their support; he could then let the emotions come to the surface and be grieved.

Within a short time after this, the couple felt a renewed sense of connection and stopped therapy. It was a profound lesson to the therapist that it was crucial to allow a patient to grieve—and to express his or her grief—in whatever way was effective for him or her and that sometimes there truly were no words to capture the raw feelings; they just needed to be felt. The therapist's role in this case was to recognize and respect the patient's need, to be willing to just be there as a silent support while the patient grieved, until the patient could once again find words. It was a good lesson that sometimes less is more and that simply asking for a description of a patient's physical experience can be less threatening and more effective than asking them to verbalize their feelings.

CULTURAL DIFFERENCES IN BEREAVEMENT

Having children is an expectation that crosses all cultures, and there is no question that infertility and perinatal loss cause emotional anguish for all. Grief for reproductive loss is universal; there are no ethnic, religious, or cultural differences in how couples feel when they are unable to have a child as they had hoped. Differences in *how* one expresses his or her grief, however, may be based on the practices of each individual's particular cultural heritage. Equally important is an understanding of the woman's role in her society. The pressure on women to produce offspring varies across cultures, and often it is the woman who gets blamed for childlessness, whether it is her "fault" or not. There may be serious consequences for those women who cannot have children, such as divorce, abuse, or infidelity (Hynie & Burns, 2006).

Knowledge of cultural norms and a woman's social role in her culture is crucial for the clinician in determining the course of treatment. If the therapist does not know what the customs are in a client's specific culture, it is perfectly acceptable to ask and be educated by the client. Treatment methods with patients of diverse cultures may or may not need to be altered. What is crucial is that the therapist is aware of the cultural expectations and interpretations of loss, so that he or she is respectful of however the patient needs to grieve. It is also vital for the therapist to be aware of his or her own personal views. Each person sees the world through his or her own cultural lens, and it is impossible to completely step out of one's own set of standards and assumptions. To help couples through the grief process, sensitivity to the similarities and differences of the patient's values to one's own values is essential.

It is equally important not to make assumptions about a client's belief system based solely on his or her race or ethnicity. Children of immigrant parents, for example, are bicultural, with their feet in two, sometimes opposing, worldviews. How much they have acculturated and blended into their current social structure will vary from person to person. They may alternate between beliefs, depending on the particular situation, falling on family traditions in one instance while pursuing convictions from their new culture in other circumstances. Mental health professionals need to listen for what may seem like contradictions in the patient's value system, to help him or her sort through the differing perspectives.

A client's concerns about ethical and moral conflicts are often expressed during infertility, when the desire to use assisted reproductive technology (ART) clashes with religious or cultural beliefs. This can be exceedingly painful. Because most societies see childlessness as an aberration, the expectation is that couples will marry and bear children. The rituals and practices of one's religion can provide support and comfort during difficult times, yet, because many religions do not support the use of reproductive technology to create life, infertile couples may find themselves caught between the pressure to procreate and the prohibitions of their particular value system. ART may be deemed unnatural and therefore unacceptable. Often the desire to have children is so great that it overrides whatever religious bans against technology exist, but this can add a layer of guilt and anxiety to an already stressful situation. How should a Catholic patient, for instance, manage frozen embryos, when abortion of any kind is taboo? Or how can an Islamic couple reconcile their wish to use egg donation when their religion dictates that ART is only acceptable if it involves the genetic material of both the husband and wife? These present terrible quandaries for couples who are committed to their faiths and yet desperately want a child.

When a perinatal loss occurs, parents may turn to religious customs or cultural mores for guidance, but others may find themselves lost without prescribed ways of dealing with a miscarriage or stillbirth. Until recently, for example, parents who had a stillbirth in the United States were given a death certificate but not a birth certificate. Many parents, in a grassroots effort, pushed for legislation to receive a birth certificate as a symbolic acknowledgment of their child, and now several states have enacted laws to issue such certificates (Lewin, 2007). The disturbing juxtaposition of death when a new baby is expected is something that everyone would prefer to ignore, but, by not legitimizing the experience, parents are left even more at a loss in their grief.

Pregnancy termination of a much-desired baby is one of the most painful situations for a couple, whether or not they have struggled with infertility. Although some genetic anomalies make the decision to terminate obvious, others are less clear-cut. The most common genetic condition for which women are screened is Down syndrome (DS; Geller, 2004). Both infertility and the incidence of DS rise with a woman's age, increasing the possibility of facing a termination. Any couple groping with the decision to terminate a longed-for pregnancy goes through agonizing doubts, but infertile couples have the added worry that this may be their only chance to have a child. Moral and ethical values are put to the test; some parents opt for early termination, whereas others decide that ending the pregnancy is not a choice, in spite of the diagnosis. Either way, these patients need support in their decisions. It may be challenging for the therapist as well; independent of one's own personal values, the role of the mental health professional is to help patients navigate this difficult decision and grieve the loss.

For some, pregnancy termination may conflict with cultural or religious doctrine. For example, in the ultra-Orthodox Jewish community, pregnancy termination is forbidden after the 40th day; in most cases, in the Muslim Arab community, it is not allowed after 120 days (Zlotogora, 2002); and in Catholicism termination of a pregnancy is prohibited under any circumstances. The journey these parents take can be agonizing: Not only are they in shock that their reproductive story does not include a healthy pregnancy, but they must also reconcile medical realities with fundamental beliefs about life and death as well as church doctrine. The decision-making process includes thinking about the life of the affected child, the welfare of other children in the family, and concerns for one's partner and oneself (Korenromp, Page-Christiaens, van den Bout, Mulder, & Visser, 2007). It is important for mental health clinicians working with this population to know that, regardless of culture or religion, women who choose to terminate a pregnancy because of a fetal anomaly may grieve just as intensely as those who spontaneously lose a pregnancy (Zeanah, Dailey, Rosenblatt, & Saller, 1993).

Gloria and Bill, for example, were naturally devastated when their amniocentesis confirmed that their third child had Down syndrome. After much agonizing, they decided that it would be best for their family to terminate the pregnancy. Following the procedure, Gloria was overwhelmed with grief, guilt, and shame. Even when her pastor and therapist validated her decision, even when she "knew that God had forgiven her," she continued to suffer, torturing herself with self-judgment. Gloria felt unable to be truthful with anyone about her loss, maintaining the "lie" that she had miscarried. This is a common reaction; many clients would rather lie than confront what may be a hostile reaction about termination from family or friends. This added to her sense of guilt and, consequently, she felt even more isolated and ashamed. If grieving a miscarriage is already disenfranchised (Doka, 1989), then mourning the loss when one has chosen to terminate is even less publicly recognized and acknowledged. Although relieved following the procedure, Bill understood Gloria's pain, but he felt helpless in his efforts to comfort her and to have family life go on as usual. He was uncomfortable lying to his other children and felt stuck between respecting her needs and theirs.

In working with this patient, the therapist recognized that Gloria's difficulties had more than one source. If it was purely a religious conflict, it might be expected that a blessing from her church would provide relief, but it did not; something else must be going on. Gloria focused her guilt and shame on her perception that she had chosen to terminate the pregnancy not to spare her child undue pain and suffering but because she did not want to handle it. She felt self-centered and selfish. The therapist asked Gloria if she had ever felt this way before. Gloria immediately blurted out that she had felt this way her whole life. She described how her mother always used to call her selfish and relied on Gloria for support when she felt depressed. Her mother continued to turn to Gloria for help, and Gloria felt unable to say no. Indeed, Gloria overidentified with her mother's neediness, such that she had her mother sleep over whenever Bill was away on business.

It emerged in therapy that Gloria's continued attachment to the unborn child was complicated by her own separation conflicts with her mother. She came to understand that it was difficult for her to attend to her own needs under any circumstances, that her depression and lifelong guilt kept her tethered to a chronic state of self-sacrifice and martyrdom. Even though her decision to abort was only partially derived from her own anxieties about raising a handicapped child, she focused all of her emotions on her own "selfishness." The therapist reframed Gloria's decision to terminate the pregnancy as a *selfless*, not *selfish* act. She focused on Gloria's concerns for her other children and, in essence, not only gave her permission to acknowledge her own personal limits but stressed how important it was to respect those limits, so that she did not "burn out" in caring for her other children. As Gloria made a cognitive shift in her interpretation of her actions, she came to see it as an act of love, of protection and sacrifice, not only for the child who would have been born with multiple disabilities but also for her other two sons. She realized that she had not chosen these events, that they were traumas that had befallen her, and that she did not need to blame herself. Most important, as she gained psychological autonomy from her mother, she recognized that her needs were legitimate and that it was not selfish to attend to those needs. Each year, on the anniversary of the termination, she lights a candle and says a prayer for her unborn child. She views him as being with God, safe and happy. In this way, she was finally able to reconcile her decision to abort with her religious beliefs and her own self-concept.

HELPING PATIENTS GRIEVE A REPRODUCTIVE LOSS

Validation

Patients have a great need for validation of the trauma that has happened to them, whether they are struggling with infertility, have had a perinatal loss, or, as all too often occurs, experience both. Previously, bereavement models treated these losses as nonevents, but over the course of the past several decades, there has been a significant change in recognizing the importance of validating these incidents (Bennett et al., 2005; Capitulo, 2005). The therapist can assist by listing and labeling the various losses that patients experience—including, but not limited to, the loss of the imagined or real baby, the loss of identity, the loss of fitting in with peers, the loss of adult developmental tasks, and the loss of the reproductive story—to confirm that a significant trauma has taken place. Giving clients the opportunity to talk about their infertility or pregnancy loss *repeatedly* and to discuss the meaning of the loss in the context of their life is a large part of the healing process. In this way, the therapist can facilitate grieving by helping patients legitimize the loss and the understandable, and inevitable, impact of the event.

Creating Rituals

Because there are so few standardized rituals for a perinatal loss, many individuals and couples don't know what to do and may look to the mental health provider for suggestions. Clinicians can make concrete suggestions and ask clients what makes sense to them. It is helpful for clients to hear what different people have done and how others have chosen to use traditional rituals or to create new ones for themselves.

Some will choose to have a funeral at their place of worship; others will create their own memorial service. These may include personally meaningful ceremonies such as planting a tree, setting off balloons, writing to their child, or lighting candles. It can also be adaptive for a couple to choose to do nothing. Again, this does not indicate that they are not grieving but, rather, that they opt for a less formalized expression of their grief. It is vital that clinicians demonstrate acceptance of the couple's decisions without criticism or judgment.

Although there are few recognized rituals for pregnancy losses, there are virtually none for the losses of infertility, but it can be very helpful to establish some. One couple, for example, agreed to have dinner out each time her unwanted menses came, not as a celebration but as a way of staying connected. The couple acknowledged that even if they didn't focus directly on "the baby issue," these dinners were helpful. Spending this time together not only acted as a catalyst for communication but also forced them to focus on what they *did* have, rather than on what was missing. Other couples may recognize their monthly loss by going for a walk together, buying flowers, or lighting a candle. Given that infertility often elicits chronic feelings of helplessness, partaking in a ritual can help couples feel more in control, that they are doing *something*. Creating a ritual for a pregnancy or baby that never was validates the reality of a loss that is so intangible.

Psychoeducation

Teaching patients about grief, and about the unique aspects of reproductive grief, is also helpful. Because there are so few guidelines, the therapist is often put in the role of educator, especially when there are differences in grieving or coping styles that are causing conflict for the couple. Because each person in the dyad may handle his or her grief very differently, they often misunderstand each other. The clinician can normalize disparate reactions as typical, but varying, grief responses to infertility or pregnancy loss. A study that taught bereaved men and women to cope in ways opposite to their normal gender roles was associated with lower distress (Schut, Stroebe, de Keijser, & van den Bout, 1997). Although participants in this study were bereaved widows and widowers, it seems feasible that this would help reproductive patients as well.

Ultimately, what is important for mental health practitioners to remember is what they must help patients remember: There are no right or wrong ways to grieve, no time lines, and no "shoulds." The variation in the intensity, timing, and expression of grief is enormous (Bennett et al., 2005). Just because someone does not show his or her feelings in traditionally expected ways does not mean that he or she is not grieving. What can become most painful for the bereaved is external pressure to hurry up and finish grieving. In the rush and bustle of daily life, our culture seems to have little tolerance for the time it takes for parents to mourn a reproductive loss. The clinician can and should "give permission" to grieving parents to take the time they need to fully process their loss or losses. This can be accomplished by reminding clients of what is normal in the grief process. Using a psychoeducational approach to teach clients about grief and mourning can be very helpful in that it normalizes grief reactions, especially if clients are feeling pressure from friends or family to "get over it."

SUMMARY

A reproductive loss is one of the most difficult experiences for an individual or couple to bear. Not only has a real or wished-for child been lost, but feelings of hope for and dreams of the future have gone terribly off course. Grieving is essential, but *how* one grieves is determined by many factors: feelings of attachment, ethnicity, religion, social mores, and gender. Mental health practitioners can help facilitate grieving for individuals and couples alike. Validation of the experience as a real trauma is key; so often these losses become minimized in an effort to "get back to normal." Also essential is an understanding of the different, but equally legitimate, ways that people tend to grieve these losses. Not only does the clinician provide support, but he or she also assists in helping clients rewrite their reproductive story to incorporate their loss or losses and pursue new endings.

6

IMPACT OF REPRODUCTIVE CHALLENGES ON INTIMATE RELATIONSHIPS

Infertility and pregnancy loss clearly have a huge effect on the individual: Self-esteem plummets; social relationships falter; questions about one's identity and role as a man or woman arise. But reproductive loss is not just an individual trauma: The strain on the couple's relationship can be profound. Although many couples—whether heterosexual or same-sex—feel that their experience with reproductive trauma brings them closer together, others grapple with feeling alone in their desperation. Because each member of the couple is dealing with this crisis in his or her own way, they may not be able to support each other or meet each other's needs. When one considers that there are two reproductive stories that have gone awry, two means of coping with this loss, and two separate time lines of grieving, it is not surprising that even the best of relationships bow under the weight of this struggle.

This chapter explores how the personal coping style of each partner and the loss of control over this arena of their life impact the couple's feelings about each other. We address both heterosexual issues as well as those unique to the gay and lesbian community. Additionally, this chapter focuses on individuals who choose to become parents without a partner. As with gay and lesbian couples, although not necessarily infertile, this population must seek alternative, often medical, means to create a family. Whatever the family configuration, there are obstacles and issues to deal with; there may be medical, legal, financial, and societal hurdles to overcome. This chapter addresses some of the challenges faced by each group when becoming parents and the therapist's role in assisting them through the process. Strategies for how the mental health clinician can help people sustain and nurture their relationships, both during the crisis at hand and afterward, are suggested.

HETEROSEXUAL COUPLES: GENDER, COPING STYLES, AND COMMUNICATION

Historically, infertility and pregnancy loss have been thought of as a female problem. Women have been blamed for reproductive difficulties: Sometimes they have been held responsible because of physical issues (e.g., uterine anomalies, fallopian tube obstruction) but also, in the past, they have been faulted for psychological reasons (e.g., possible ambivalence about becoming a mother; Benedek, 1952; Deutsch, 1945; Leon, 1990). The responsibility placed on women is likely due to the physical act of carrying a pregnancy as well as cultural gender roles and expectations. Although gender roles have become less differentiated in developed Western cultures, with men taking on more child-care responsibilities, the primary role for men is still viewed as that of provider, whereas women continue to be considered the family caretaker (Berg et al., 1991).

When statistics are examined, however, the myth that women are chiefly responsible for fertility issues is found to be false. The data reveal that men and women share the diagnosis of infertility equally, with about one third of the cases attributed to male factors, one third to female factors, and, for the remainder, either both members of the couple have subfertility or the problem is unexplained (American Society for Reproductive Medicine, 1996–2009). Interestingly, even when the etiology of infertility has been identified as male factor, women *feel* the brunt of the responsibility for the lack of conception (Wright, Duchesne, Sabourin, Bissonnette, Benoit, & Girard, 1991). In spite of the infertile couple's diagnosis, studies suggest that women take on more guilt and blame than their partner (Beaurepaire, Jones, Thiering, Saunders, & Tennant, 1994; Greil, Leitko, & Porter, 1988). Furthermore, regardless of the source of infertility, women reported less marital and sexual satisfaction (Lee, Sun, & Chao, 2001). Again, this may be due to gender-specific socialization, with women's need for family as role defining being more powerful than men's.

What if one person has been diagnosed as having "the problem"? He or she may feel damaged and guilty and may worry that the partner will blame him or her as well. In fact, it is common for the infertile person to worry that his or her partner may want to end the relationship entirely (Andrews, 1984). "If I can't give him (her) a baby," the thinking goes, "why would he (she) want to be in this relationship?" The affected individual may even act out—by being explosive or by having an extramarital affair—to create a self-fulfilling prophecy (Menning, 1976). This behavior may be viewed as a test of commitment: "Will he (she) continue to love me, in spite of my erratic behavior—and infertility?"

After a pregnancy loss, feelings of guilt are common as well. Many women assume responsibility for the demise of their pregnancy, as if their actions, or inactions, were to blame. They may be haunted by self-reproach: Was it the sip of wine I had? The plane flight to a conference? Did I carry too many groceries? Exercise too much? The list of self-incriminating questions is endless, all in an effort to make sense out of the loss. Men, too, can feel guilty: One man was convinced that he "caused" the demise of his wife's second pregnancy. He noted that he helped out a lot more during the first, successful pregnancy but was less available for the second, thus putting her more at risk.

Even if the blame is irrational, many people find it comforting to assume some cause for their loss, rather than to have no reason at all. Attributing a cause to the pregnancy loss—even when it is inaccurate—allows a couple to feel that they can avoid repeating the behavior in the future and helps them regain a sense of control. "The doctor keeps telling me that nothing I did caused my miscarriage, but I don't really believe him," explained one woman. "I am perfectly healthy, and so was the fetus—things don't just happen for no reason. In retrospect, I wish I hadn't been so set on going to the mountains for vacation—maybe the altitude caused the problem." The doctor's reassurance and the fact that many women are pregnant above sea level did not assuage her guilt. Although she was incorrect in her interpretation of the events, her self-blame was easier to handle than the free-floating anxiety of having no explanation.

Factors That Influence the Experience for Men and Women

There is little doubt that infertile women, or women who have had a reproductive loss, have greater levels of anxiety and depression than women who are able to conceive and give birth to a healthy child (Merari, Chetrit, & Modan, 2002). But do women suffer more than men? Cultural expectations and gender role socialization promote the notion that women do feel more pain than men during a reproductive crisis, and some research supports this notion, noting that women have higher distress levels than men at such times (Andrews, Abbey, & Halman, 1991; Greil et al., 1988; Newton, Sherrard, & Glavac, 1999). Greil et al. (1988) found that, whereas women get "thrown for a loop" emotionally, men feel disappointed but not devastated; whereas women's identity is threatened, men are more concerned about their spouse's happiness and want to have life return to normal.

Men's struggles with reproductive events, however, are just as legitimate as women's, although they may be expressed differently (Berg et al., 1991; Butler & Koraleski, 1990). Men report aspects of infertility treatment (providing sperm samples, worrying about finances) to be particularly stressful (Mahlstedt, 1985). Although a woman's involvement in an infertility workup, for example, is largely medical (she is beset with invasive and physically painful procedures, requiring more demands on her time), men's participation is largely sexual in nature. Providing a sperm sample on demand in a doctor's office causes performance pressure, anxiety, and embarrassment for many men. "One doctor we saw used a lab across the street in the hospital," explained one man. "I had to go over there, do my thing, and then carry it back across the parking lot to the office. I felt ridiculous, and was sure that everyone knew what I was doing." In addition to the sexual exposure and embarrassment, male infertility tests and procedures can also be extremely anxiety provoking. Surgical procedures involving the penis or testicles often are terrifying to a man, reminiscent of early childhood castration anxiety. Often, men will joke about such matters with other men, in locker rooms or while playing sports, but it can be extremely difficult for a man to talk about his fears directly, with either his partner or a therapist. Again, the use of a psychoeducational approach can be very helpful: The therapist can explain, for example, that "many times, men feel: uncomfortable discussing such things. . . . feel like they are the only ones . . . are ashamed, scared or upset by their thoughts . . . " These are very common and completely normal thoughts and fears; men may need to be reassured that it is okay to talk about them.

With the lion's share of attention focused on his partner, a man may feel excluded from the process. He may feel pressure to support his partner; consequently he may suppress his own negative feelings, which in turn may lead to depression and/or a sense of helplessness. As discussed in Chapter 5, men's grief is often internalized, potentially resulting in long-term emotional consequences (Puddifoot & Johnson, 1999; Toedter et al., 1988).

Nonetheless, a woman's struggle may intensify because of the physical nature of these events. Her ongoing monthly cycle is a continual reminder of what is missing. Although men may pay less attention to a woman's bodily fluctuations, women are acutely aware of every hormone shift, every ache or cramp, especially as she is trying to conceive. The physicality of a pregnancy loss requires a woman's body to undergo enormous stress, and it can take months for her to feel like herself again. Some patients have described a literal feeling of emptiness, a hole where the baby should have been. If the loss was at or near term, her body will respond as if a baby had been born and will produce breast milk. This is one of the most traumatic pieces—both physically and emotionally—of the loss.

Age is also an important factor to consider; as women get closer to reaching the end of their reproductive life span, they report higher levels of distress when a loss occurs (Berg & Wilson, 1991). It makes sense that, as their biological options decrease with age, their anxiety about becoming a parent increases. Although it is common knowledge that women have a biological clock, many couples are less aware that there are declines in men's fertility with age as well. Age affects men's sperm quality, hormone levels, and erectile functioning and may increase the risk of miscarriage because of genetic abnormalities (Fisch, 2009). Studies suggest that conception rates decline as men reach their late 30s (Dunson, Baird, & Colombo, 2004) and that it can take 5 times as long for men over 45 to impregnate their partner, compared with men who are less than 25 years old (Hassan & Killick, 2003). More studies are needed to determine the effects of age-related infertility on men's emotional state.

Age also plays a part in the social timetables regarding parenthood (Daniluk & Tench, 2007). If peers are having children, couples may feel added pressure to have children around the same time. One infertile couple noted with enormous sadness that most of their friends were having second children, while they were still struggling to have their first. Age may also decrease the availability of alternative options for parenthood, such as adoption (Daniluk & Tench, 2007). Couples may feel an urgency to adopt because of age restrictions; they may be forced into considering other parenting possibilities before they are psychologically ready.

Differences in Coping

Because of the intensity of the emotions and the extended length of time couples may spend in a crisis mode, their usual methods of coping with stress get stretched to the limit. The emotional wear and tear can cause communication to break down to such an extent that a member of the couple may question the very basis of the relationship itself, asking, for example, "Is this the same person I fell in love with? Do I really want to have a family with him or her? Will our relationship be able to sustain itself without children? What if he or she leaves me because I can't have a child?" These questions add even more angst and insecurity to an already vulnerable situation.

Not only does each member of the couple have to come to terms with his or her own trauma but he or she must also deal with how the partner is coping. For example, when stressed, some people manage their feelings by withdrawing; they may need to process their feelings privately. Others tend to seek out support and have a need to talk about and sort out their emotions openly. Some may lash out in anger, whereas others may internalize it. Some people feel more in control of their anxiety if they plan for and research all possibilities, whereas their partner may believe that dwelling on issues before they arise is a waste of time or will somehow jinx what they are doing. Some do better when they have a contingency plan in place (i.e., researching adoption while continuing with in vitro fertilization [IVF] treatments), whereas others need to see Plan A to completion before they can consider Plan B. And although some seek to garner more control over their life by taking action, others may need to disengage. Drowning oneself in work or destressing in front of the TV both provide some sense of escape and may seem adaptive, but what often happens is that one partner may misunderstand the other's coping style and misinterpret it as not caring. Although particular responses in coping may be helpful for the individual, they could have a deleterious effect on the couple's relationship.

Just as there are differences in how each gender grieves a reproductive loss (as discussed in Chapter 5), coping styles seem to split into typical male and female patterns. Women tend to turn to others for help through this emotionally difficult time. Because women are in more overt emotional distress, they may seek out psychological treatment more than men (Daniluk, 1991), and they are more willing to attend support groups than their partners (Lentner & Glazer, 1991). Additionally, women tend to avoid social situations that might be emotionally stressful, including attending baby showers, going to shopping malls, visiting with friends who have children, or attending family gatherings. Men, on the other hand, may throw themselves into work or other projects in which they can feel productive and effective. They are more likely to cope by keeping their feelings to themselves, partly in an effort to protect their mates from more emotional pain (Williams, Bischoff, & Ludes, 1992), and to feel as if they should support the needs of their wives over their own (Mahlstedt, 1985). Although unintentional, conflicts can arise because of these differences in coping styles: Whereas women have a need to talk to their spouses about these issues, men find that talking about them increases their level of stress (Valentine, 1986), and men's avoidance of such discussions leads wives to believe that their husbands don't care.

Clinical observation suggests that some men completely defer to their wives when it comes to making reproductive decisions. Many men, in their effort to please and be supportive, will go along with "whatever she thinks is best. After all, it is her body." In yielding to her wishes, however, men not only give away their power, but they also put their partner in the uncomfortable position of feeling alone in this complex decision-making process. She may misinterpret her husband's lack of opinion as a lack of commitment on his part to have children and may feel as if she is trying to start a family all by herself. It was found that if the decision to pursue infertility treatment was one-sided, there was less marital satisfaction both during and following treatment (Pepe & Byrne, 1991).

Discussing this in the therapy session can be most beneficial to the relationship; not only will the woman feel less resentful, but when the man becomes a more active participant in the decision-making process, he will feel less out of control. The mental health practitioner can help bring to light how each person manages his or her feelings and how this may affect the other. It is essential for the therapist to help couples identify their own and their partner's coping style, to allow a deeper understanding of how each other deals with loss, how each makes decisions, and how to avoid misinterpreting each other's behavior.

As the following cases illustrate, misconstruing a mate's behavior can lead to increased alienation. To open dialogue and communication, couples must recognize that there are no right or wrong ways to manage their stress, that they may have different reactions to the exact same event, and that their needs at any given moment may be poles apart from each other.

When the therapist first met them, Jake and Corinne had been struggling with infertility for 3 years, with a nonspecific diagnosis. They had tried intrauterine insemination (IUI) twice, did an IVF cycle that failed, and were preparing for their second IVF procedure. Jake is a former military officer who now works in the defense industry as a civilian. Corinne is a child psychologist. In the first session, Jake expressed concern that Corinne had seemed very depressed recently, that "she had lost her spunk and all she wanted to talk about was getting pregnant." Corinne acknowledged that she found it very helpful to talk about her feelings, both with Jake and with friends; she felt frustrated that Jake was so private and self-contained: "It's almost as if he doesn't care." When the therapist turned to Jake for his perspective, he responded immediately, exclaiming that "I would not be here if I didn't care, but I'm just not so worried about it." He went on to comment that he was a very optimistic person, felt confident that they would eventually get pregnant, and got frustrated with what he perceived as Corinne's negativity.

"Life will pass us by if we're not careful," he admonished her. "What's the point of dwelling on being sad? It won't help and we miss out on so much else. If I sat around moping all the time, I'd be depressed too." The therapist took this opportunity to ask Jake how he handled his stress about the infertility. "I try to stay active," he said. "If I keep busy, I don't think about it as much." Jake spent his weekends playing sports and helping his father remodel the basement. The therapist used this information to highlight their coping styles. She pointed out that although Jake and Corinne cope differently, each style is legitimate. The problem came in misinterpreting the other's behavior rather than recognizing it as a way of coping. She also pointed out, however, that the hours Jake spent on physical activity and the project with his father filled a secondary need as well: avoiding his wife's emotional state. She noted that when Jake was off pursuing these activities, Corinne felt alone and abandoned. "He never puts me first," Corinne interjected. "There is always something more important for him to do than be with me."

Corrine went on to express her fears that she was pushing Jake away and had tried to "be strong for him." Jake was shocked to hear that his wife was worried about his commitment to her. "Sometimes I stay away because I think you don't like me anymore," he lamented. "It seems that all you care about is a baby." In turn, Corinne was surprised. The therapist emphasized that this was why it was so important that they explain their feelings and behaviors, to avoid misinterpretation and hurt feelings. She encouraged the couple to view each other with compassion and to ask directly for clarification if they were feeling upset by their partner's behavior.

In another session, Corrine arrived after a difficult day at work. The therapist encouraged her to talk about it, knowing that the stress from her job may well be intensified by the infertility trauma. Corinne lamented that her job was a daily reminder of her failed reproductive story. She found it almost impossible to keep her feelings at bay, especially when she saw children whose parents seem incompetent in caring for them. "It's unbearable to watch parents who fail to do even the basic nurturing. I am constantly modeling how to talk to these kids, how to comfort them. It's always there—the feeling that if this were *my* child—how different it would be." When she got home, she needed support and reassurance from Jake, to help her decompress and process the day, but this had become really difficult for Jake. He admitted that when he sat and talked with his wife, he ended up feeling worse, because no matter how hard he tried, it didn't seem to make her feel better. "I wish she was back to the way she used to be." Corinne's sadness left Jake feeling inadequate. He knew that "just listening" *should* be the best way to help his wife, because it showed her that he cared and was interested in her feelings, but it never felt like enough. "I think if it was just once in a while I could handle it, but this is every day. Maybe I just don't know how to do it right," he said, revealing yet another example of his sense of incompetence.

The therapist empathized with Jake's frustration at not feeling like he could adequately help his wife, and Corinne reassured him that when he did sit and listen, she felt much better. But the therapist also explained to Corinne, "that just as she needs Jake to be willing to talk with her, he needs time to himself. Because he deals with his emotions more internally than she does, he needs private time to work through his experience." The therapist emphasized the importance for Corinne not to take this personally but to recognize his absences as his way of coping. In these sessions, the couple learned to negotiate their communication and their time. Jake agreed, for example, that they could talk every day, but Corinne agreed to set a time limit so that Jake would not become overwhelmed. They also acknowledged that there would be exceptions to this, that some days Corinne might need more time and other days Jake might need extra time to himself. They both agreed not to take these times personally and felt they could manage these exceptions; because the rest of their communication would be more structured, both felt they would be understood and supported. Understanding each other's coping style allowed the couple to deal with the stress of the upcoming IVF cycle in a much more constructive way.

Negative Impact on a Couple's Sexual Relationship

Sexual intimacy is one of the most significant aspects of a couple's relationship that is affected by reproductive trauma. Although sexuality is only one facet of a relationship, for couples who have had difficulties conceiving or who have had a pregnancy loss, feelings about their sexuality, fertility, and relationship merge. Sex turns into a chore, a means to an end, rather than an expression of love and desire. It becomes difficult for couples to separate baby-making from lovemaking, when sex feels like an assignment. The sexual act itself may serve as a reminder of what is missing from the couple's life; the additional stress that couples feel may produce impotence and/or decreased libido (Berg & Wilson, 1991).

All spontaneity is lost when sex is on a schedule and "prescribed" by doctors. The anxiety caused by sexual intimacy, brought on by the stresses of infertility treatment, is apparent in both men and women (Peterson, Newton, & Feingold, 2007). Peterson et al. (2007) speculated that men's anxiety may be more related to sexual performance, whereas, for women, the anxiety has more to do with the outcome of the sexual act, that is, becoming pregnant. However, the pressure the couple feels regarding their sexual intimacy can occur even when the couple is not actively engaging in sex. Women may measure and chart their temperature on a daily basis to time ovulation; awakening to a beeping thermometer is enough to quell anyone's sexual appetite. The medication prescribed for ovulation control and stimulation can make a woman feel bloated and unattractive, further diminishing her desire for romantic encounters. Additionally, couples are often advised to wait 36 to 48 hr after intercourse before engaging in it again, to replenish sperm (Greil, Porter, & Leitko, 1990), which interferes with spontaneity. Men may feel controlled by their partner's monthly ovulation cycle (Beaurepaire et al., 1994) and resent having to perform on demand. Indeed, having to provide a sperm sample at a specific time, under pressure, can lead to temporary impotence. Clearly, making a baby in the sterile environment of a doctor's office is not the way it was supposed to be. When a couple's intimacy gets turned into clinical records shared by physicians and medical staff, they lose all sense of privacy. It's no wonder the romance in the relationship diminishes or even disappears.

Berg and Wilson (1991) examined couples' marital and sexual satisfaction across stages of infertility treatment. During the 1st and 2nd years of treatment, they found that although individuals experienced depressive symptoms, their sexual and marital relationships remained adequate. When couples reached the 3rd year or beyond, however, not only did depressive symptoms increase, but marital and sexual satisfaction reached their lowest point. Thus, the chronic stress and repeated sense of failure have a cumulative effect, which has a negative impact on the couple's sense of intimacy.

Pregnancy loss can have a similar impact on the couple's sexual relationship. The loss of self-worth and diminished body image can lead to a decrease in libido for women (Boxer, 1996; Serrano & Lima, 2006). Guilt or self-blame for the loss may also lead clients to deny themselves pleasure as a form of self-punishment. They may feel additional guilt if they do allow themselves positive experiences. Furthermore, for reproductive patients who have miscarried, the very thing they desire—a baby—comes with the threat of another loss, creating a kind of approach–avoidance struggle within the individual. Sex after a loss may be emotionally painful, because, as with infertility, lovemaking and baby-making are intertwined. Sex after a loss, with the purpose of getting pregnant, may fill both partners with anxiety and fear of yet another failure. Both members of the couple may feel guilt in having disappointed their partner: She in not being able to get pregnant or carry a pregnancy to term and he in not being able to impregnate her. He may also worry that he has caused her physical and/or emotional pain if the pregnancy fails. It is important for the mental health practitioner to address these issues, because couples can confuse their conflicts with intimacy with problems in the relationship.

Sometimes, couples need permission to take a break from trying to conceive (of course, only if it is medically acceptable to do so). They may feel as if their time is running out, and even a short break may feel like they are losing opportunities. But taking some time off can do wonders for the relationship. When couples allow themselves to reconnect without the pressure of conception, they may be able to renew their feelings for each other. Therapists can play a vital role in helping couples restore their bonds to each other, sexual or otherwise. Helping couples communicate their feelings about intimacy at this time—their frustrations, their dissimilarities in sexual desire, and their differences in coping—can regenerate closeness. Additionally, finding alternate ways for couples to express closeness—surprising each other with a gift, giving each other a massage, just holding one another—can increase intimacy, without sex.

The impact on sexual intimacy, however, can have long-term effects on the couple. Pepe and Byrne (1991) found that even 2 years after infertility treatment was terminated, the negative impact on the sexual relationship was still felt. This may be especially true if the resolution of their reproductive crisis ends in childlessness (Daniluk & Tench, 2007). During treatment, the focus of sex turned from something pleasurable to the task of procreation, and switching gears again can prove difficult for many couples. Recapturing the desire for the other, without the possibility of producing a family, can cause deep sorrow. These issues are often very difficult for couples to bring up with each other; likewise, they may have a challenging time in initiating discussion of sex in the counseling setting. It is helpful for the mental health practitioner to address these issues as part of assessing the overall health of the relationship (Daniluk & Tench, 2007). If these issues remain unspoken, the shame, embarrassment, guilt, or anger that a person is feeling may intensify. It helps if the therapist brings up the topic of sex in a matter-of-fact, normalizing way. When the therapist shows him- or herself to be comfortable with such "unspeakable" issues, it can free the couple to articulate their experience, rather than keeping it inside as a shameful secret.

Financial Concerns

The price tag that comes along with infertility treatment can be another issue that affects the quality of the couple's relationship. The cost of treatment may, in fact, force decisions about the direction a couple takes in creating their family. Although some medical insurance plans will cover a portion of the costs for certain treatments, most people have to supplement with considerable out-of-pocket sums. And there are some courses of action, such as paying for a surrogate, that are outside the realm of medical insurance reimbursement. Likewise, a couple might be torn between risking another round of IVF or putting that money toward adoption; in this way, dollar signs rather than emotional readiness may dictate family-planning choices.

The substantial costs involved—for what everyone else, it seems, can do for free—add to the feelings of loss and inadequacy. Savings may get depleted, home purchases may be delayed, existing homes may get mortgaged to the limit, and other acquisitions may get put on hold indefinitely. In fact, couples may feel that everything in their life is on hold—from buying new carpeting, taking a much-needed vacation, or going back to school. Patients feel uneasy, and sometimes guilty, if they spend money on something other than medical treatment. Complicating an already difficult issue, couples often need to borrow considerable sums of money and may turn to their families for help. Asking for financial assistance can be rife with emotional baggage. Already in a compromised position, clients may feel even more regressed having to ask for money, as if they were teenagers again, dependent on their parents. Couples may feel obligated to their parents in uncomfortable ways: If the parents are paying, or helping to pay, for a procedure, do they have a right to make decisions about it or to know the step-by-step details of the process? This may feel like another intrusion into the couple's private life. And what if the procedure fails? Will the couple feel an increased pressure because of parental involvement? Additionally, what if both sets of grandparents-to-be are not able to contribute equally? Discomfort may arise for patients if their respective parents have differing ability and/or willingness to give.

In general, deciding where and how to spend money can be difficult interactions for couples. When the emotional stress of infertility and loss of well-being is added to the mix, tension about money may be magnified. Just as each person has a different style of coping, there are varied and wide-ranging approaches to dealing with money. One partner may have a more conservative style of spending money, whereas the other may be more willing to take a risk. One may have more confidence that they will be able to earn enough to pay off debt, whereas the anxiety of spending huge sums of money may be too much for the other to bear. Couples may also disagree on what is important to spend money on. The emotional value placed on their future family can take on new meaning as they come to grips with financial limitations. One member of the couple may be willing to chance all on yet another round of in vitro, for instance, whereas the other may focus on the odds of success and determine whether this is a wise financial decision. Clearly, this can create a great deal of conflict within the couple; often, decisions about treatment are made on emotional grounds, and casting such decisions in terms of financial wisdom makes many people uncomfortable. It may feel as if it minimizes how important that child is to the couple, or it may feel as if they are "buying" a baby when they must pay so much.

Just as it is helpful for the therapist to explore the couple's individual and shared reproductive stories, it is also very important to help the couple articulate the complexities of their "financial stories." Differences should be approached in a spirit of understanding and compromise. When a person knows why his or her partner feels a certain way, it is easier not to take the reactions personally and to have compassion for the other's anxiety. In turn, a focus on how each person can compromise, meeting the other in the middle, defuses the sense of impossible stalemate. In fact, negotiating compromise is perhaps one of the most useful skills a therapist can help couples learn.

SAME-SEX COUPLES

Reproductive technology has opened pathways to parenthood not just for heterosexual couples but also for gay and lesbian couples. A "gayby" boom (Dunne, 2000) is occurring, with increasing numbers of same-sex couples having children. Controversies and myths regarding gay and lesbian parenting abound; concerns about the child's emotional welfare, social acceptance, development, and sexuality are often cited. One of the "arguments" against gay and lesbian parenting is that the parents will influence their child or children to become gay. This assumption has been shown to be false: The sexual orientation of parents—whether heterosexual or homosexual—has little bearing on the child's sexual orientation (Bailey, Bobrow, Wolfe, & Mikach, 1995; Green, Mandel, Hotvedt, Gray, & Smith, 1986; Golombok & Tasker, 1996; Patterson, 1992). Another myth is that children of homosexual parents will be teased or bullied more than their peers parented by heterosexual parents and that this will lead to psychological difficulties. Studies have debunked this misconception as well; it was found that children growing up in same-sex families were no more likely to suffer from social or emotional problems than those of heterosexual families (Dunne, 1999; Golombok, Spencer, & Rutter, 1983; Green et al., 1986; Patterson & Redding, 1996). As with children growing up in a gay male household, having lesbian parents does not have adverse effects on the children (Mooney-Somers & Golombok, 2000). Additional follow-up research on young adults brought up in a lesbian household demonstrated that they continued to fare as well as their counterparts from heterosexual families (Tasker & Golombok, 1997).

An ironic result of the societal homophobia so prevalent in our culture is that many gay people who wish to be parents have unconsciously internalized these very same homophobic or heterosexist ideas: The belief that they do not have a right to be parents or could not possibly be good parents because of their sexual orientation (Sophie, 1987; Parks, 1998). In the past, many gay men and lesbians did not think it was possible for them to become parents; they questioned whether it was a legitimate thing for them to even want. They may have accepted the idea that parenting is not something that same-sex couples have the right to desire, even if they had always wanted to have children. Sadly, this can undermine the confidence of people who would otherwise be proud of their parenting skills. Because of this self-doubt, they may feel the need to prove themselves as a parent (Parks, 1998).

Lesbian Couples

In order for a lesbian couple to build a family, they may choose to adopt, have heterosexual intercourse, or use donor insemination (DI). With DI, lesbian couples, just as heterosexual couples who are dealing with male factor infertility, must decide whether to use a known or unknown donor. McManus, Hunter, and Renn (2006) noted the pros and cons of using either a known or unknown donor for lesbian couples. With a known sperm donor, the couple may worry about ongoing involvement with the donor as coparent. Fear of a custody battle with the donor trying to take the child away may lead many lesbian parents to choose an anonymous donor. On the other hand, many lesbian couples choose a known donor so that their child or children will have more of a sense of their biological roots. Some sperm banks have a program in which the donor agrees to have his identity revealed after the child turns 18 years old (Chabot & Ames, 2004). This allows the child, if he or she wishes, to know more about his or her genetic heritage. If this feels like it will come too late in the child's life, the option of using a known donor may be more appealing. A clear understanding of what the relationship with the donor will be, if any, and legal documentation of the rights of all parties involved are clearly necessary prior to insemination. Depending on the openness of the couple, the child or children may actually have a positive relationship with their genetic donor and benefit from having a male role model (McManus et al., 2006).

Another challenge lesbian couples face is the determination of who the biological mother will be. Sometimes there is a clear-cut choice of who becomes pregnant, based on age, fertility, health, or the desire to experience pregnancy and birth. Some couples decide that the older partner should attempt pregnancy first, followed by another pregnancy for the younger partner. Another option is to use an IVF procedure, with fertilized eggs of one partner (with donor sperm) transferred into the other partner. This way one woman has the biological connection (the nonpregnant partner) while the other carries the pregnancy and gives birth (McManus et al., 2006). This allows both to feel that they are contributing as parents and are jointly involved in their child's conception.

In some cases, however, which partner should become impregnated is not obvious, and they may both be vying for the possibility. This can cause strain in the relationship, evoking a sense of competition (Drescher, Glazer, Crespi, & Schwartz, 2005). The therapist can act as a sounding board if this presents a problem. If one of the partners discovers that she has fertility problems in the process of trying to conceive, it is possible that the other partner will try to become pregnant instead. Although this seems like a reasonable solution, it can stir up feelings of sadness and loss for the infertile partner. Infertile women often complain how difficult it is to see other pregnant women; it is a reminder of their own loss and sense of failure. Imagine then how painful it may be to have a partner who is pregnant, if the biological piece of pregnancy and birth was highly desired. After the birth, the nonbiological mother may feel as if she is not a "real" mother, leading to feelings of disenfranchisement (Hadley & Stuart, 2009). Although it is not easy, the therapist can facilitate discussion of the full range of feelings in order for the couple to heal and move on to parenting.

Some lesbian couples with children may divide housework and child care equally, whereas others may stick to more traditional gender roles, with one parent the primary wage earner and the other the primary caregiver. The research of Hadley and Stuart (2009) suggests that these roles may be formed because of the identification with parental figures in one's own family of origin. It is here where the individual's reproductive story and the earliest sense of parental identity are formed. Although some may idealize the egalitarian nature of lesbian mothers, others point to a power dynamic inherent in all relationships, same-sex or heterosexual (Hadley & Stuart, 2009). What is important for the therapist to keep in mind is that not all lesbian relationships are the same: There are those that tend toward a more equal division of labor, whereas others divide their roles in a more traditional "mother–father" manner.

The issue of biological parenthood in same-sex couples becomes critical should the couple break up or in the case of death of the biological parent. Same-sex marriage is a highly controversial, politicized, and volatile issue. During the first draft of this chapter, same-sex marriage was illegal in the United States, except for Massachusetts, California, and Connecticut; the legality in California, however, after some 18,000 marriages have taken place, has since been revoked. From a legal standpoint, because same-sex marriages are not nationally recognized, the laws that protect the rights of divorced heterosexual families are virtually nonexistent for gay or lesbian households. Second-parent adoption is an arrangement to legally protect the parental rights of the non-biological parent should the relationship end. It allows same-sex couples to adopt their partner's biological or adopted children, but it is also not recognized in every state and can be contested by a third party (Hare & Skinner, 2008). Thus, the nonbiological parent's rights are legally vulnerable should the relationship dissolve.

As in most cases involving dissolution of adult relationships, it is the children who suffer most. Even if the nonlegal parent was highly committed to raising the child and had been a parent for the child's entire life, the non-childbearing lesbian has limited legal rights (McManus et al., 2006). Without legal parental status, the parent–child relationship of the nonbiological parent may be tenuous (Zicklin, 1995). One of the most important factors in analyzing these cases is *intent*. In other words, at the time of conception, whom did the involved parties intend to be the child's parents? If in a same-sex couple it was agreed that both partners were committed to raising the child together, then their rights as parents, whether biologically related or not, should be maintained. Another factor, *behavior*, has to do with who cares for and is responsible for the child. Concrete behaviors, such as participating in the insemination, living with the child, supporting the child, and holding the child out as her own, are all ways that the courts perceive parenthood (Hare & Skinner, 2008).

As noted in Hare and Skinner (2008), several cases have gone before the California Supreme Court, which ruled in favor of the child's best interests and granted each party involved parental rights. In *Kristine v. Lisa* (2004), for example, the two women obtained a prebirth agreement defining them both as the "joint intended legal parents" of the child and that in the event of a breakup, they would each still maintain parental status. Furthermore, the baby girl's last name was a hyphenated joining of both Kristine and Lisa's surnames. This provided a clear *intention* of the couple's initial understanding. Lisa, the nonbiological mother, was present at the insemination, provided Kristine emotional and financial support during the pregnancy, paid for the child's medical insurance, and took care of the child. Thus her *behavior* also indicated that Lisa acted as the child's parent. After the couple separated, Kristine wanted Lisa's status as "second mother" to be terminated. The California Supreme Court, however, recognized Lisa as the "presumed father" and argued that the prebirth agreement needed to be honored and that the child could, in fact, have two mothers (Hare & Skinner, 2008).

Another interesting case involved two women in a lesbian relationship, one of whom donated her ova to her partner, with the *intention* of raising children together. In *K.M. v. E.G.* (2004), K.M. agreed to donate her eggs to E.G. with the specific idea that they would parent together. They registered as domestic partners and selected a sperm donor together—again showing intent and behavior—but because of a consent form for ovum donor that K.M. signed, she waived her rights to a relationship with any child that was born using this procedure. This is not atypical; donors customarily do relinquish their rights to the child. In this case, however, because of the couple's previous relationship, the California Supreme Court found that the contract did not apply to lesbian couples when one partner donates her ova to the other. The court recognized that motherhood could be based on both the genetic relationship as well as through giving birth. Thus, it was established that a child could have two mothers—one gestational and the other genetic— provided that there was a committed relationship between the two women (Hare & Skinner, 2008).

Although same-sex marriage and parenting are becoming more recognized socially as well as legally, there is still a long way to go. Mental health clinicians should be aware of the issues that same-gender couples undergo in their attempts to become parents and in the homophobic struggles they may face. Who "the mother" is in a lesbian relationship can be challenging to define; helping patients better understand their roles and the needs of their child or children is vitally important. It is also imperative to keep in mind the child's experience in the potential dissolution of the parent's relationship.

Gay Male Couples

For better or worse, society's stereotype of a primary parent is that of "mother" (Friedman, 2007). Historically, it has been a rare occurrence for men to choose to become parents, either on their own as a heterosexual or gay male, or as part of a committed homosexual relationship. More common is for a gay man to have had children from a previous heterosexual relationship. Although in the past gay men may have longed to be fathers, their options were limited; they may have sought out an arrangement with a woman to coparent as a way to fulfill this need. Presently, although homophobic stigma is still a reality, it is more accepted and easier for male partners to make the conscious decision to build a family through either adoption or surrogacy.

Domestic adoption laws regarding same-sex couples vary from state to state. Currently, in every state except Florida, gays, lesbians, and bisexuals may adopt as individuals. Although many states expressly approve legal adoption by gay male couples,[1] others may support it (with approval by lower courts) but have no explicit laws (Lambda Legal, 2008). Because there is no national policy legalizing same-sex adoption, gay men may feel forced to choose between living in a legally sanctioned state and one that is not (Lobaugh, Clements, Averill, & Olguin, 2006). Clearly, it is not always possible or even desirable to move away from job, family, or support system for the express purpose of adoption. International adoption also has challenges for homosexual couples; it is controversial and not accepted in most countries around the world. Because of this, gay men and lesbians who wish to adopt internationally may decide to present themselves as single parents, so as not to face discrimination (Friedman, 2007).

The controversy surrounding the legality of same-sex adoption ostensibly has to do with overall concerns for the child. As noted earlier, the fear that a same-sex couple will influence their child's sexual orientation is unfounded (Bailey et al., 1995; Green et al., 1986), as is the worry that children raised in a homosexual household will be bullied and teased more than others (Dunne, 1999; Golombok et al., 1983; Green et al., 1986; Patterson & Redding, 1996). Although these children fare as well as their peers, some gay couples steer away from adoption for fear that birth parents will prefer a heterosexual couple for adoption. They may also worry that adoption agencies will consider them a "last resort" and offer them children with mental and/or physical problems (Lobaugh et al., 2006).

As an alternative to adoption, gay men may turn to surrogacy. Whether they choose traditional surrogacy, in which the surrogate uses her own eggs with the man's sperm without sexual contact, or gestational surrogacy, using a donor's egg, the man's sperm, and a third-party surrogate, they will use the same assisted reproductive technology (ART) procedures as infertile heterosexual couples. For many men, the reasoning to use a surrogate rather than to adopt parallels the feelings of heterosexual couples. They want a biological connection with the child and a sense of control. It may be difficult for a

---

[1] California, Connecticut, Delaware, District of Columbia, Illinois, Indiana, Iowa, Maryland, Massachusetts, New Jersey, New York, Pennsylvania, and Vermont.

couple to decide which partner should be the biological father. Men may choose to alternate, using sperm from one partner on each insemination attempt, or to use sperm from both in a single IVF cycle (Friedman, 2007).

Just as with lesbian parents, gay men may also question "who does what" in caring for their child; defining their roles may be challenging. Because gay male parenting is a relatively new phenomenon, there are few role models for men to follow. It may be that one partner will take on the role of primary care-giver, but, because gay men often do not keep to gender stereotypes, the role as a parent may be more adaptable and less limited than their heterosexual counterparts. It also may be that their parental tasks evolve and develop naturally over time, as it does in most families. Gay men may turn to the mental health professional for help in the process. They are forging new territory within a world that is often not tolerant of any aberration of the traditional family model. They need support, not only in dealing with their sexual orientation but also for decisions regarding conception and family planning.

Despite the stereotyped expectation that women are best suited to the role of mother, clinical experience with both heterosexual and gay men underscores that the process of attachment and bonding to one's child is every bit as meaningful to men as to women. This is illustrated by Chris, a lawyer, and Michael, owner of a retail business, who employed an anonymous surrogate to carry their child. They had been partners for 8 years when the idea of having children came up. At first they were tentative about it: Would their families accept their choice, would their child suffer because they were not in a traditional family? The more they investigated their own feelings as well as how other men coped with parenthood, the more they knew they had a lot to offer a child. With great excitement and nervousness, they carefully researched available surrogates and chose a woman who lived in another city. Despite the physical distance of the surrogate, Chris and Michael felt very involved in the pregnancy and began preparations for their baby right away, painting the nursery and thinking about names. When the surrogate miscarried at 12 weeks, they were all devastated. The surrogate felt that she had let them down, and Chris and Michael were grief stricken that their baby had died. It is crucial for therapists to understand and appreciate the deep attachment that occurs in the transition to parenthood, regardless of gender or sexual orientation, and to recognize that men have reproductive stories that go just as deeply as women's stories.

SINGLE PARENTS BY CHOICE

Although there have always been parents who have *had* to raise their children single-handedly, as a result of divorce or the death of their partner, this section focuses on those who consciously choose to be solo parents. In

Western culture, there are both men and women who are choosing to "go it alone," and, although the number of men who become single parents by choice (through adoption or surrogacy) is growing, statistics are few. These men often face difficult obstacles: The cost of surrogacy is high, surrogates and donors may not think of single men as suitable parents, and birth mothers may see them as their last choice (Navarro, 2008).

Single women who choose to become parents have a relatively easier time than their male counterparts, and there is considerably more research on them. Perhaps society is more accepting of single mothers than single fathers because of the expectation that motherhood is part of a woman's role and identity. A single mother by choice has been defined as "a woman who decided to have or adopt a child, knowing she would be her child's sole parent, at least at the outset" (Single Mothers by Choice, 2007). Statistics for this subgroup are hard to determine because "choice mothers" are lumped into the same category as other single mothers (i.e., unwed teens, divorced women). The numbers, however, are definitely growing: Single Mothers by Choice (an international support group founded in 1981 by Jane Mattes, CSW) reported that new membership in 2005 was nearly double what it was in 1995 (Egan, 2006). Single mothers by choice are demographically similar: They are usually in their late 30s, well educated, professional, and financially secure (Mannis, 1999; Murray & Golombok, 2005a; Weinraub, Horvath, & Gringlas, 2002). They are acutely aware of their biological clock ticking and feel that time is running out. Although many claim they would have wanted to parent with a loving partner (Mazor, 2004)—which can be assumed to be part of their original, ideal reproductive story—they no longer feel they can wait.

Women who choose to become single mothers have the option to adopt, have a casual sexual relationship with a man specifically to become pregnant, or use DI. Although DI has traditionally been used for couples dealing with male factor infertility, there is a growing trend for women who elect solo parenthood to use it. The majority of single women who want a child choose DI, because they don't want to have casual sex in order to have a child, are concerned about health risks (HIV or other sexually transmitted diseases), don't want to deceive a man, and don't want a man involved (Murray & Golombok, 2005a).

Solo mothers by choice have been categorized as a unique subgroup of single-parent families (Weinraub et al., 2002), because there are marked differences between "choice families" compared with other single-parent families. Research on fatherless families—those created because of death or divorce—has consistently shown that children pay the price. These children tend to do less well at school and have more emotional and behavioral problems than their peers who have two parents (Murray & Golombok, 2005a). The performance of these children, however, may have less to do with the lack of a father and more to do with other environmental factors. For example, women who are single mothers *not* by choice often have less financial means available to them (Mannis, 1999). The lower socioeconomic status of these women was found to be the greatest factor in the underachievement of their children (McLanahan & Sandefur, 1994). Because the choice mothers are usually economically secure, their children do not face the same struggles as the "nonchoice mothers."

Another reason children in single families have poorer adjustment than children in intact families may be because of the emotional traumas to which they were exposed. Children who have lived through their parent's separation or divorce are often subjected to fighting and conflict between their parents. The emotional distress children feel—and the subsequent psychological problems they experience—have more to do with their parents' breakup than with single parenthood. In fact, separation and divorce affect children's behavior more than if their parent had died (McLanahan & Sandefur, 1994). The distinct difference between children raised by mothers who choose single parenthood and others is that these children are not exposed to divorce or loss. As a unique group, the past research on single-parent families should not be generalized to the choice families (Murray & Golombok, 2005b).

One might assume that raising a child and working to support a family on one's own would be an enormous and stressful undertaking. Murray and Golombok (2005a, 2005b) conducted two recent studies on the differences between solo DI mothers and their married counterparts who used DI because of male infertility. They measured the psychological well-being of the mothers, the quality of the mother–child relationship, and the child's development. Interestingly, the results revealed that the solo DI mothers and their children were fairing quite well. In the first year of the child's life, solo DI mothers did not differ from married DI mothers in their adaptation to parenthood, and there were no significant differences in levels of anxiety or depression. The authors concluded that the lack of a father did not have an effect on the emotional state of the solo DI mothers (Murray & Golombok, 2005a). This trend continued through the child's second year of life as well. In fact, the solo DI mothers took greater pleasure in their child, and, as a whole, the children were noted to have fewer emotional and behavioral problems (Murray & Golombok, 2005b).

The researchers also noted that 93% of solo DI mothers planned to tell their child about the donor conception. They were committed to honesty in the relationship with their child and did not want to promote family secrets. Additionally, they were more likely to be open with other people about their conception. In contrast, only 46% of married DI mothers planned to tell, whereas 30% decided not to let the child know. This discrepancy may have to do with the stigma of the father's infertility. Solo DI mothers are making a conscious choice to use DI, not because they have struggled with their own or a partner's male infertility. On the other hand, DI was not the first choice of the married mothers; they had chosen DI because male factor infertility was preventing conception. They may have more feelings of shame because of the infertility and may want to protect the father's feelings (Murray & Golombok, 2005a, 2005b).

Although there is much focus on the difficulties that gay, lesbian, or single parents have, there is also evidence that suggests that nontraditional families often create a whole community of loving adults, a "village" so to speak, who participate in the raising of the child or children. Research on lesbian couples, for example, indicates that these families receive a great deal of support not only from their families of origin but also from their social network, especially other lesbian mothers (Parks, 1998). A case in point is of Ann and Joan, a committed lesbian couple, who recently gave birth to a baby boy by DI using sperm from their close friend, Marty. Marty is engaged to a woman with a 3-year-old child, and the two couples view each other as "family." In addition, Joan provides child care for her neighbor's 5-year-old daughter, who loves "Aunt Joanie." Somehow, all the members of this cast manage to maintain appropriate boundaries and clear recognition of their roles. The children feel loved and supported, and the tasks of parenting are made easier for all by the wide net of support the adults provide one another. There have been similar research findings that highlight the creative ways in which single mothers join forces for support (Hertz & Ferguson, 1997; Mannis, 1999). Stacy, a single-by-choice mother, describes how she teams up with other single mothers for support, for friendship, and for help in child raising. These families, as non-traditional as they seem, are actually not unlike families from the past, in which children may have had relatives who lived nearby or neighborhood friends who would act as extended family and pitch in to help with child care.

SUMMARY

Couples not only struggle with their own reproductive trauma and loss of their individual reproductive story, but at the same time must cope with each other and respond to what may be vastly different coping styles and grieving patterns in their partner. Regardless of family configuration, individuals and couples contend with medical, societal, legal, and psychological challenges that can be overwhelming and can affect their intimate relationship. It can be helpful for the therapist to encourage the couple to share their reproductive story with each other and identify the various ways in which they manage their stress. This can do much to alleviate any misunderstandings and hurt feelings that can arise at such times.

The confluence of the rise of ART at a time in history when the idea of *family* is not limited to the traditional mother–father–child model has opened avenues to parenthood for gay men, lesbians, and single men and women, as well as heterosexual couples who are dealing with infertility and pregnancy loss. Mental health practitioners should not only be aware of the particular issues these families face but also be sensitive to their own biases, if any. Often, gay or lesbian couples will seek help from a gay or lesbian therapist, but not always. As with all reproductive patients, it is imperative that therapists, regardless of their own sexual orientation, remain neutral and supportive as their patients traverse these parenting options.

7

AT A CROSSROADS: FACING THIRD-PARTY REPRODUCTION AND ADOPTION

The issues that individuals and couples contend with when faced with infertility and/or pregnancy loss are many. As discussed, there are numerous losses that must be grieved, internal personal struggles and identity issues triggered by the trauma to resolve, and potential conflicts within the couple's relationship itself that need attention. One such crisis point for clients is when the possibility of having their own, shared biological child has come to an end. After years of trying, couples must decide what path, if any, to take next. In the midst of grieving the dream of a genetically shared child, couples must face one of the hardest decisions they will ever have to make. The myriad possibilities can be both a blessing and a curse; there are more options for family building today than ever, but the array of choices may leave couples feeling overwhelmed and uncertain about what to do next. Although any of the options can be rewarding and satisfying, it requires much thought and soul-searching to reach a point of resolution.

The choices include

- donor technology—ovum, sperm, or both, with either a known or anonymous donor;
- embryo "adoption"—the couple uses embryos that have been frozen and donated by another couple;

- surrogacy—either gestational (an in vitro fertilization [IVF] process, where an embryo implants in the surrogate's uterus; the embryo can be made in any number of combinations—using the mother's eggs, the father's sperm, or with donated eggs and/or sperm) or traditional (the surrogate uses her own eggs with the father's sperm);
- adoption—either domestic or international; and
- a child-free life.

Because their original reproductive story is no longer a reality, patients must decide what parts of it they are willing to "rewrite" and what they will be comfortable with in the long run. They need guidance in this uncharted territory, as many questions that tap into moral, spiritual, and cultural beliefs are raised by the advent of the available scientific technology. The therapist can help individuals and couples identify the most salient pieces of their story—what they are able to relinquish and what they are hoping to keep intact—and the compromises they are then willing to make. For example, is the experience of pregnancy the most important part of the story? If so, then donor technology would be appropriate. If the genetic connection to the child is primary, then surrogacy using the gametes of both parents could be considered. If raising a child is the guiding principle, regardless of whose DNA is used, then adoption becomes viable. These are difficult things to think about, and often these ideas are being considered for the first time. In fact, patients may begin this process absolutely convinced that they would never consider donation, adoption, or surrogacy, only to find themselves opening to the idea when facing the reality of their situation. As one couple described their dilemma, "We need a blueprint for figuring out the next best option for us."

Using a psychoeducational approach, therapists can encourage patients to "try on," for however long is needed, the various possibilities—that is, their new possible selves (Markus & Nurius, 1986)—to see what fits the best. Just as one takes a car for a test drive to see how it handles, or tries on a dress to see if it fits, clients can consciously fantasize about the various scenarios, to help them identify how they might feel and what they worry about. They can make a more psychologically informed decision if they ask themselves such questions as: How will it be to hold a baby who is not genetically connected to me? How will family and friends react? Will we be accepted as a family in our place of worship or our community? What will it be like to tell the child the story of his or her birth? The therapist can recommend that couples think about their reactions to these kinds of questions in the present day as well as 5, 10, or 20 years from now. Trying out different possible selves with the future in mind gives patients an additional perspective, helps them step outside of the present crisis, and allows them to see that there are viable solutions.

The mental health professional can help provide the blueprint by laying out the positives and negatives of each option, discussing the individual or couple's concerns, and assessing their response to each choice. Whether one is considering single parenthood or parenthood as a couple, it can be helpful for each person to analyze his or her feelings independently from others before coming together for discussion. This way each can express his or her feelings without censure. This is a time for brainstorming and considering all ideas and for talking about things without feeling that the discussion ties them into one point of view. If clients can agree to put it all out on the table—all their fears, concerns, and desires—doing so can help them accept their ultimate decision.

When working with couples, it is common for therapists to see one person taking a more passive position in the decision-making process. As previously discussed, we have found that men, in their effort not to make demands or put pressure on their partner, will leave this decision of what to do next up to her. Invariably, this leads to misunderstandings and resentment. She feels as if she alone is responsible for family planning and her partner is less invested in the outcome. Addressing this dynamic in therapy allows the couple to open the dialogue once again and come to a joint decision.

It is important for therapists to realize that they may have their own wishes for their patients' reproductive futures. It can be difficult for a therapist working with a couple considering embryo donation, for example—or any alternative form of family building—to be as direct and honest about the realities of the risks and limitations as they need to be. Therapists may unconsciously worry about scaring their patients away from a decision, if they are forthright about the risks, and may hold back, especially if they are invested in their patients becoming parents. Chapter 8 explores the complexities of therapists' reactions to their clients' decisions. As discussed, it is foremost that therapists consider their clients' needs first.

The couple's reaction to the options before them can also give the therapist insight into their sometimes unspoken, often unconscious, feelings. Until faced with these decisions, each member of the couple may not have even realized what would be acceptable to him or her; it is only when forced to move in a new direction from their original story that these feelings emerge. This chapter addresses each option available for couples and the psychological struggles entailed in coming to grips with these choices.

USING DONOR TECHNOLOGY

Donor insemination (DI) is the process by which a woman is impregnated using the semen from a man who is not her partner. Although it is primarily used by married couples with male factor infertility, lesbians and single women who want to have a child also use this procedure. Additionally, gay men may use DI to create a family using a surrogate. Lazzaro Spallanzani (1784), an Italian biologist, performed the first successful mammalian DI using a dog, but it was not until the 1930s, when the ovulation cycle of women was fully understood, that DI became a viable option in humans. By 1941, more than 10,000 women had become pregnant using DI (Bullough, 2004); since World War II it is estimated that over a million babies have been conceived in this way (Orenstein, 1995).

By comparison, the use of ovum (or oocyte) donation (OD) is relatively new. The first baby born using an egg donor was in 1984, following advances in IVF technology (Lutjen, Travinson, Lecton, Findlay, Wood, & Renou, 1984). The procedure is much more complicated than DI in that both the donor and the recipient must coordinate their menstrual cycles using medication (stimulating ovulation and egg production in the donor and suppressing it in the recipient) and then use IVF to transfer the fertilized embryos into the recipient's uterus (in most cases using her partner's semen). OD is widely used by older women whose eggs are no longer viable and by women who have diseased or damaged ovaries because they are cancer survivors or because of other genetic anomalies.

For many women, the experience of pregnancy and childbirth is an aspect of their reproductive story that they hope not to forfeit. Using donor technology to become pregnant, whether ovum, sperm, or both, is a wonderful option for them. Not only are they able to hold on to this portion of their story, but they may also derive a sense of mastery over their otherwise unsuccessful attempts at conception. But whereas the medical procedures involved in donor technology have become somewhat routine, the emotional issues that accompany the technology are complex. Many questions emerge for clients as they wrestle with this choice, and it is common—and normal—for feelings to flip back and forth in considering the "right" thing to do:

- Is it unethical to go to such lengths to create a child when there are children already in need of homes?
- Is using a donor tampering with nature?
- Does it go against religious mores?
- Will the partner who is not genetically connected feel differently about the child than the parent who has the genetic link?
- Will the couple be able to withstand a possible pregnancy loss?
- Is it better to use a known or anonymous donor?
- If a known donor is used, will the relationship with the donor change and if so, how?
- If the donor is anonymous, on what basis is the choice made? On the basis of physical features? intelligence? health? family history?

- What will other people think?
- How does one tell the future child where he or she came from?
- And perhaps most important, has the client grieved the loss of his or her own fertility sufficiently enough to be able to truly accept and feel comfortable with the use of a donor?

Although recipients are usually not mandated to consult with a mental health professional, it is strongly advised that they do, even if only for one session. Recipients, caught up in the excitement of taking action and moving forward, sometimes ignore the complexities of using a donor. The mental health professional can serve as a guide in bringing up issues that may have a psychological impact on the recipients in the present as well as in the future. Not only is it important for clinicians to raise these questions with their patients, but helping their patients find answers that are personally meaningful to them is key to the ability to feel confident in their decision.

It can be frustrating or anxiety provoking for the therapist to observe potential recipients waver as they grapple with this decision, wanting them to take action and move on. Indeed, their ultimate choice may not be what the therapist would have chosen; it is vital for the therapist to remain neutral and help clients figure out what is right for *them*. It is also essential for therapists to remember that, at the same time individuals and couples are trying to come to grips with moving forward in this process, they are grieving—the loss of their own biological offspring, the loss of sharing this with their partner—in essence, the loss of their original reproductive story. This is extremely important for therapists, patients, and medical staff to recognize. Although the availability of donor technology is a gift that allows parenthood, it also comes at a price: the final acceptance that one's own fertility is not viable. The following case example typifies the struggles patients face in considering the use of a donor.

Janine, 37, and Ryan, 40, have been dealing with unexplained infertility for 7 years. Because they were relatively young when they began trying to conceive, their doctor had them do four cycles of intrauterine insemination (IUI) before he recommended IVF. They then endured five IVF cycles, including two that were conducted back to back, in the hope that the hormonal overlap would aid conception. Having decided to stop their efforts to create a biological child, they are now at a crossroads in their journey, trying to decide whether to try egg donation, pursue adoption, or remain child-free. Janine, although exhausted from the physical ordeal of treatment, wants to try using an egg donor, longing for the experience of pregnancy and birth. "I have given up so much already," she laments. "This would be a chance to have at least part of the experience I dreamed of." She nevertheless feels ambivalent about egg donation and wonders if it is somehow wrong to artificially create a child from donor eggs, who would never otherwise exist. Ryan, on the other hand, is ready to adopt. He feels it would be less unfair—that if one of them could not have a genetic tie to the baby, then neither of them should. Neither can yet envision choosing to remain child-free, although Janine sometimes feels so overwhelmed and afraid of failure that she "just wants to chuck the whole thing, move downtown and be child-free yuppies."

Janine and Ryan, like so many other couples at this juncture, are not only trying to deal with their emotions but are also grappling with religious, cultural, and moral beliefs. Many cultures and religions do not approve of third-party reproduction, feeling as if it is a violation of the traditional hetero-sexual union of man and woman. The notion of adding a third person to the couple's relationship can cause uneasy feelings because it defies conventional ideas of family bonds. Some couples worry about sexual fantasies they or their partner may have about the donor. The involvement of a third person in the relationship may feel morally distasteful, akin to an extramarital affair (Thorn, 2006).

Although Janine and Ryan don't feel they are breaking with their religious beliefs, they have many moral and ethical concerns. They worry that they are being selfish if they choose to use egg donation, citing the benevolence and altruism of adoption. They feel guilty about putting their own needs before those of others, knowing that "there is a child out there" who could benefit from a "good home." Some couples, especially those who have experienced a miscarriage or pregnancy loss, worry about the uncertainty of pregnancy and the possibility of another loss, whether donor technology is used or not. For this reason, many couples prefer adoption, noting that there will definitely be a baby at the end of the road. On the other hand, some have an overwhelming fear that the birth parents will change their minds or that the child will have significant developmental or health issues.

Ryan had many concerns about using an egg donor. If they chose OD, he feared the day that someone would comment on how much their child looked like *him*, and not *her*, and he dreaded what that might do to Janine. "Resemblance talk" is a common social phenomenon: People often comment on the resemblance of children to their parents, and, in a sense, this legitimizes the child's belonging to that family (Becker, Butler, & Nachtigall, 2005). Becker et al. (2005) found that the issue of resemblance is something that all parents of donor offspring—whether sperm or egg—find challenging. Not only were couples concerned about how resemblance talk might affect their child, but some experienced it as a painful reminder of their own infertility and lack of a genetic link with their child. The therapist reminded Janine and Ryan that it is very common for children to look like one parent and not the other and that siblings often look nothing like each other. She described one family who had one adopted dark-haired child and two blond biological children: Their relatives "forget that Annie is adopted, because she looks just like her aunt"—also a dark-haired sibling to two blonds. Their therapist also reassured them that, as children get older and develop the habits and mannerisms of their parents, whom the child looks like becomes less of an issue. Resemblance then becomes more a function of behavior than looks.

Another related emotional issue that couples wrestle with when considering donor technology is the attachment to the child. Ironically, clinical experience has indicated that it is usually the parent who *will* be genetically related who worries about their partner's attachment to the baby. Ryan, for example, expressed his concerns that Janine—as the nongenetically related parent—would feel less connected with their child. Janine, however, was not concerned about her attachment, citing that she would be carrying the baby and bonding through the course of the pregnancy. In fact, the reason that she was leaning more toward OD rather than adoption was that she wanted to be able to have Ryan's child.

In other families, however, the nongenetic parent may have a lot of anxiety about whether he or she will be able to truly love and connect to a baby born from donor gametes or whether the baby will love him or her as a "real" parent. These patients may benefit from some discussion about the nature of attachment. The therapist can explain that the kind of attachment between a parent and baby is far more powerful than any other connection and has nothing to do with genetics. Attachment with a baby has more to do with the daily care, love, and nurturance that a parent gives—and the reciprocal loop of satisfaction that occurs between the parent and child—when a baby becomes soothed. Parents of premature babies, for example, also worry about attachment to their infant if they have to be separated at birth for medical reasons, and yet they form passionate bonds with their babies despite that traumatic separation. It can also be helpful to remind patients that the reproductive story begins long before a baby is created or born and that this early emotional attachment precedes *any* pregnancy.

Pointing out the research that has been done on donor families can allay some of the fears clients have as well. For example, Golombok et al. (2004) compared families who had a child conceived by gamete donation (50 DI and 51 egg) with 80 natural-conception families. The researchers found that the families who used a donor had more positive relationships with their children, with greater emotional involvement, than the natural-conception families. Similarly, research on DI found that attachment between the father and child was not negatively affected by the lack of a genetic tie (Golombok et al., 2002). The parent–child relationship may, in fact, be strengthened because of the great lengths couples took in becoming parents; they truly don't take it for granted, and they have a greater appreciation for parenthood and of their children.

ANONYMOUS VERSUS KNOWN DONATION

Once couples make the decision to use a donor, the question arises as to whether they will seek out an anonymous donor or use someone they know. In most cases of DI, the donors are anonymous, whereas it is much more common for OD to be interfamilial or from a friend (Thorn, 2006). The advantage of using a donor from one's family—a sibling, cousin, niece or nephew—is that it allows the recipient to retain some genetic link to the child. Bartlett (1991) found that the motivation to use a family member as an OD fell into four categories: (a) the longing to have a baby, (b) the desire to experience pregnancy, (c) the hope to give their partner a genetically related child, and (d) their own desire to have a genetic link to the child. Using a friend or other identified donor may also alleviate anxiety of the unknown.

Although the recipient may feel more secure with a known donor because it eliminates the mystery of the donor's medical, social, and educational history, it may raise other issues concerning the donor–recipient relationship. A study that examined the relationship of a recipient with a known donor found that, although many recipients felt that the relationship with the donor would become closer, some reported that they would feel indebted to the donor (Bartlett, 1991). The relationship may take on new dimensions when a child, who is connected to both the donor and recipient, is added to the mix. Boundaries may get blurred: Will the donor feel entitled to make decisions about parenting? Will the question of resemblance create awkward moments for parents and donor alike? What happens if a falling-out occurs? These are important issues for the recipient, donor, and therapist to consider, because the impact on the relationship can have a direct and long-lasting effect on the donor, parent, and child's life.

Using an unknown donor presents its own challenges: Primarily, on what basis does one make this choice? In many countries, donors are selected for the recipients by the doctors or clinics on the basis of matching physical characteristics (Thorn, 2006), but in the United States an essentially free market exists in choosing a donor. Although sperm banks have been in existence for quite some time, the phenomenon of using an unknown ovum donor has given rise to agencies that act as egg brokers. Many medical clinics also recruit donors, and the Internet is yet another avenue recipients may research in order to find a match. Because this is a largely unregulated market, recipients should be advised to thoroughly investigate the source of the donor before making a commitment.

In general, the recipient will receive information about the donor, including family background, medical history, psychological history, academic interests, personal hobbies, and why they have decided to donate. In addition, current photographs as well as baby pictures of the donor are usually available to view. For many, the donor's physical looks, intelligence, and personality are the most important factors to match with the recipient (Greenfeld & Klock, 2004). Other factors that recipients look for are health (mental and physical), race, education level, and hobbies (Sachs & Burns, 2006). Clinical experience suggests that a general resemblance to the recipient is usually desired; many hope that the child will blend into the family, with physical differences not readily apparent. Some worry that they are being too vain, wanting a child who looks like the recipient, but, as discussed previously, the issue of resemblance can help the family feel more cohesive. Additionally, depending on their reproductive history, some recipients may want a "proven" donor: someone who has either successfully donated before or is already a parent. It can be exceptionally traumatic when a couple endures the emotional, physical, and financial stresses of using a donor, only to have it not work because of problems with the donor's eggs or sperm.

A large and growing movement is afoot to change the way donor anonymity is addressed. In the past, donor identity was kept completely confidential; it was thought best to keep this a secret to protect both the child and the parents from feeling different (Shanley, 2002). More recently, however, awareness of the child's needs and rights to know his or her biological origins has pushed thinking toward eliminating donor anonymity. Many countries have passed legislation allowing information and/or contact with the donor when the child reaches legal age (Thorn, 2006). Both the Human Fertilisation and Embryology Authority of the United Kingdom and the Assisted Human Reproduction Agency of Canada have recently eliminated all donor anonymity and compensation and have created a centralized donor registry (Sachs & Burns, 2006). Some fear that "open" donation will diminish the number of people willing to donate. Others worry that the child's relationship with the recipients, or social parents, will be negatively affected, but, as the vast literature on adoption informs, this is not generally the case. Abolishing anonymity may allow the child to know that his or her birth was due to a real, and as is most often the case, altruistic person.

Also under current debate is the matter of compensation for gametes, especially for egg donation. Sperm donors have traditionally been paid a nominal fee, but because of the scarcity of ovum providers as well as the far more complicated procedure to procure eggs, the practice of paying egg donors large sums of money has become the norm in the United States. Advertisements for egg donors in college newspapers are common, and the offer of thousands of dollars in payment may be quite alluring to students, who would not only like to help an infertile couple but who also are concerned about paying off student loans (Shanley, 2002). Even more important, although the American Society for Reproductive Medicine (ASRM) has created specific guidelines for the screening and compensation of donors, there is no formal legislation in the United States that legally protects either the gamete donor or the recipient if medical complications occur or the recipient does not become pregnant.

DECISION TO TELL

The use of donor technology is a grueling process: Decision after decision must be made. Once couples make the choice to go the donor route, they must then decide whether to use a known or anonymous donor, each of which, as we have discussed, has its pros and cons. If they opt for an anonymous donor, the deliberation over what donor characteristics to choose begins. Hours, days, and weeks may be spent pouring over photographs and descriptions supplied by their doctor's office, donor agency, or the Internet. In addition to all of these considerations, couples must also grapple with what might be the most anxiety-provoking decision—that of disclosure. Whom do they tell and what should they say? Should they tell their families, friends, or coworkers? Is it okay to tell her parents and not his? What happens when they all get together for a holiday and someone slips and spills the beans? If a couple does tell someone in confidence, how will they feel if and when the information is leaked? Some report that they have told no one—except they had to tell a friend because they needed help with a shot, or they had to tell their boss because they needed extra time off—without realizing that their "secret" may get out. Many couples feel ashamed and stigmatized by their fertility problems, and this extends to embarrassment about using a donor as well. Some may worry that they will be judged for not adopting. Additionally some individuals struggle with their sense of identity—"Am I the 'real' mother (or father)?"—and may worry that others will question it as well. These are the concerns that haunt clients and make them debate what is best. Although some are extremely open about the experience, others are selective about sharing the information, and still others prefer to keep their procreation choices entirely private. Herein lies another issue: What if one person in the couple wants to be open and the other does not? As with any disagreement, understanding the reasons why each person feels a certain way and then negotiating a compromise is an important therapeutic task.

Aside from disclosing to others, the key issue parents face is whether to tell their child. Reasons *not* to tell include concern that the child will be confused about who his or her parents are and may fantasize about his or her "real" parent, fear that the child's development and happiness will be disrupted, and worry that the child will feel stigmatized by the conditions of his or her birth (Salter-Ling, Hunter, & Glover, 2001). On the other hand, parents who want to disclose feel that the child has an inherent right to know, are uncomfortable keeping a family secret, and worry about the potential harm to the child, should he or she find out inadvertently from another source (Salter-Ling et al., 2001). According to Nachtigall (cited in Orenstein, 2007), on whichever side of the argument parents fall, their motivation is the same: They believe they are acting in the best interest of their child. The parents' desire to protect their child from the possibility of insensitive comments from people outside of the family is often what motivates them to keep conception details secret, whereas disclosing parents are more concerned that a secret of this sort would disrupt the family dynamics of trust (Nachtigall, cited in Orenstein, 2007).

Parents also question *how* to tell their offspring. On one side, there is the "seed-planting strategy," which purports that early disclosure is best: Children grow up always knowing about the circumstances of their birth. On the other side, is the "right-time strategy," which suggests that it makes more sense to tell a child when he or she can better understand the biological processes involved (MacDougall, Becker, Scheib, & Nachtigall, 2007). Some parents feel like the right time is when the child asks, "Where do babies come from?" With either approach, parents need to understand that children may have many questions that change over time and that as they mature, they will process the information, both cognitively and emotionally, differently. Children's questions should always be answered in an age-appropriate manner: Younger children, for instance, can be told that "there is a mommy part and a daddy part" and "mommy's (or daddy's) part didn't work, so we used a part from another mommy (or daddy)." There are also children's picture books available that address third-party reproduction—making it easier for both the child to understand and for the parent to have a guide in approaching the subject (ASRM has a list of books for children, http://www.asrm.org).

So how are people to make a decision concerning a child who is not yet created? Notwithstanding individual concerns or preferences, it may be helpful for patients to know that a growing movement supports telling the child about his or her biological origins. This parallels the trend toward a more open approach to the donor's identity, as the issue of donor anonymity has come under scrutiny. Although at the present time in the United States there is no legislation in this area, the ASRM Ethics Committee has come out in favor of disclosure to children (ASRM Ethics Committee, 2004b). The report points to the need for "open and honest communication with children," and, taking the position of proponents of open adoption, suggests that telling a child sooner rather than later allows the child to absorb the information over time. Research has also supported this position; it is thought that secrecy can lead to tension within the family and that disclosure is ultimately better for the child (Van Berkel, Candido, & Pijffers, 2007). Another study of DI families noted that children who were told the circumstances of their birth had fewer behavioral problems and overall a less tense relationship with their parents

(Lycett, Daniels, Curson, Chir, & Golombok, 2004). Although the decision remains with the parents, the mental health practitioner can help parents understand the pros and cons of disclosure and help them find ways to best approach the topic with their child.

WHEN THE DONOR IS THE PATIENT

As mental health practitioners, we are often called upon to assess the psychological appropriateness of ovum donors. (Rightly or wrongly, it is not general practice for sperm donors to undergo a psychological evaluation.)[2] Clinicians need to rule out donors with severe psychological pathology, assess whether a donor will be able to follow through with keeping her appointments and following the medical protocol, and make sure the donor comprehends the medical procedure, with knowledge of the potential physical risks involved. The evaluation typically includes a clinical interview as well as the Minnesota Multiphasic Personality Inventory II or the Personality Assessment Inventory.

Emotional risks are involved as well, and the mental health practitioner should also review these with the egg donor. Because of the current state of anonymity with these procedures, it is likely that the donor will not know whether the recipient has had a successful pregnancy and birth. Many donors claim not to feel any attachment to their genetic material and do not think of it as their child; this is not surprising, given that many of the donors are young women, whose childbearing plans may be thought of as events that will happen sometime in the future. Nevertheless, donors may fantasize about what the child looks like and what characteristics of themselves might be seen in the child. To have a genetic offspring "out there" may feel very different to a young woman in her early 20s than it might feel later on in her life. She should be aware that the child or children produced from her eggs might seek her out someday. Additionally, the impact on the donor's current or future partner and/or present or future children is also something that the therapist or evaluator should discuss with the donor. Addressing these issues with the donor is not meant to dissuade her; rather, the issues need to be presented to have her full informed consent. It should be noted that men who are donors may also have many of the same feelings, but because they are not required to have a psychological screening, the data on them are virtually nonexistent.

---

[2]There are several possible reasons for this. Perhaps it is because of the more complex medical process of oocyte donation that a clinical interview and some form of standardized psychological test are used, perhaps it is because sperm donation has predated the technology and awareness associated with egg donation, or perhaps it pertains to the need for physicians to protect themselves against malpractice, given the medically complicated procedures that oocyte donation entails.

Unlike for male donors, the procedure for women donors requires taking hormones to stimulate ovulation and undergoing a medical procedure to retrieve the eggs. These procedures are not without risk: Ovarian hyperstimulation and infection are possible negative outcomes. Additionally, the jury is still out on the possible long-term effects from taking ovulation-stimulating hormones. So one of the key questions for the clinician to ask is: Why do you want to donate? Motivation for many donors is altruistic. Donors often know someone who has struggled with infertility; they report that their eggs are wasted every month, and this gives them an opportunity to help in some way (Bartlett, 1991). On further investigation, Bartlett (1991) found that about one third of the donors in her study had had a prior abortion and viewed the donation as a way of "making up" for it. Although many donors deny the lure of financial compensation, this is certainly a motivating factor for some.

If the donor and recipient are family members or close friends, then the nature of the donor–recipient relationship must be explored. The mental health practitioner should ascertain whether the donor feels coerced or obligated in any way. The history of the relationship may point to subtle pressure on the donor to agree: A younger sister may feel she was always bossed by her older sibling, a friend might feel indebted to help, or the donor may worry that the relationship will end or change in some way if she said no. If a red flag gets raised, the mental health professional should suggest that the recipient and donor rethink this decision and perhaps use an alternate donor.

EMBRYO DONATION

In undergoing IVF, there are often more embryos produced than can be used in any one cycle. The dispensation of these embryos is entirely in the hands of the couple who produced them, and very often they are used to produce a sibling child. Even so, there are more than 400,000 embryos stored (frozen) in the United States today. For some couples who do not want to use the embryos for themselves in the future, the idea that they would be discarded or used for scientific research is unacceptable; some people even view this as an abortion. There has been a growing movement, especially among certain religious groups, that encourages the donation of these embryos to other couples who are also struggling with infertility. The embryo(s) get transferred to another woman with the idea that she and her partner will give birth to and raise that child as their own. Embryo donation may be desirable if both members of the recipient couple have fertility problems and if they prefer not to adopt in the traditional way. As with egg and sperm donation, embryo donation allows the recipient couple to experience pregnancy and childbirth and to control the prenatal environment. In this sense, embryo donation can be a good solution for both sets of parents—donors and recipients.

Because embryo donation is such a new phenomenon, there has been little research to date on the child's development and how the family functions on the whole. In an exploratory study, MacCallum, Golombok, and Brinsden (2007) compared embryo donation families who had children 2 to 5 years of age and with adoptive as well as IVF families. They wanted to ascertain whether an absence of a genetic tie would influence parents' feelings of attachment and the quality of the relationship with the child. Their findings, in comparing embryo donation with IVF families, suggest that genetics plays no part in the parents' investment in their child. Whether there was a biological link or not, these parents, who went to great lengths to have children, were highly invested in parenthood (MacCallum et al., 2007).

Also of interest, the researchers found no evidence to support the notion that the experience of pregnancy (with embryo donation) resulted in a better parent–child bond than did adoption. The physical prenatal bond was not an essential element to positive parental attachment (MacCallum et al., 2007). This supports our hypothesis that the attachment to the desired, fantasized child starts much earlier than pregnancy; it begins with the development of the early reproductive story. The bond, therefore, is one that is psychological rather than physical, an important distinction for clinicians to note in helping couples reach their family-building choices.

At this point in history, adoption and even IVF have become common and acceptable avenues to parenthood. Unlike the adoption process, where parents are counseled at length and have more support available to them, parents who use donated embryos appear to be more defensive and secretive about disclosure. The hesitancy of these parents to disclose to their child was in sharp contrast to the IVF and adoption families (MacCallum et al., 2007). This may be due to the relative newness of embryo donation and the social stigma that may be attached to it. Although the children in the MacCallum et al. (2007) study did not appear to be adversely affected by their parents' secrecy, the children were quite young. Follow-up studies are necessary to see how these families fare over time. It is likely that, eventually, as embryo donation becomes a more recognized and established procedure, the need for concealment will lessen.

Many questions remain, however. Unlike egg or sperm donations, which may result in multiple half-siblings, the children created with embryo donation have full siblings, raised in different households. This is most analogous to adoption, in which siblings may be placed in different families, but the difference is that these embryos were created all at the same time. Will this affect the development and feelings of these children? Will the two (or more) sets of parents consider an open relationship and allow the siblings to meet? Will the genetic parents and their children become extended family? Will the recipient parents feel judged by the donating parents? Although the answers may not be definitive and may vary case by case, the mental health professional can assist both the recipient and the donor in contemplating these questions.

Last, when considering embryo donation, it must be remembered that, during an IVF procedure, typically the "best" embryos are implanted and the remainder frozen. These frozen embryos may or may not be of as high a quality as is optimal. Couples who choose to utilize donated embryos must recognize that they may be taking some risk that the embryos will not result in a viable pregnancy.

SURROGACY

Although the issues of using donor technology can be complicated, the psychological challenges of using a surrogate are even more so. Although a donor agrees to a procedure that is medically complex, the commitment made by a surrogate, who vows to carry and care for a pregnancy and give birth to a child whom she will not parent, is even more extensive. A donor may be committed to several weeks of involvement, but a surrogate, by nature of the time it takes to carry a baby to term, is engaged with the intended parents for months. It requires an enormous amount of trust: relying on the surrogate to take good care of herself, eat well, get enough rest, not use drugs or alcohol, and show up for doctor appointments. It also requires trust that the surrogate will part with the infant without conflict. As such, therapists are called upon to evaluate surrogates (as they are for egg donors), to ensure their appropriateness. Additionally, because of the potential impact on the rest of the surrogate's family, a clinical evaluation should be conducted with the surrogate and her partner. This allows the mental health practitioner to review the risks involved, both physical and psychological, thus ensuring that the consent is fully informed. As a requirement for a woman to become a surrogate, she must have at least one child of her own; consultation with a therapist can help the surrogate answer her child or children's questions about the pregnancy and what happens to the baby after delivery.

Why would a woman wish to become a surrogate? Compensation is understandably high, but this tends to be only a small motive for surrogates. Arlene, 31 years old and the mother of two young children, is a pragmatic, thoughtful, and caring person; her story typifies the reasons for being a surrogate. "My daughters mean the world to me; I can't imagine life without them. So when I thought about what it must be like for someone who can't have this experience, I knew I wanted to help." When Arlene first discussed this idea with her husband, who is a police officer, he was not very enthusiastic and really couldn't understand her passion. He couldn't fathom why she would want to put herself through such a physical ordeal for someone else. "When I asked him why he puts his life at risk at his job every day, he got it," she explained. "He understood the need to help and make a difference in the world."

Surrogates are used if a woman is unable to carry a baby to term; this may be caused by a disease that requires a hysterectomy (e.g., uterine cancer or endometriosis) or if the woman has a birth defect (often a result of her mother taking diethylstilbestrol, a synthetic estrogen, ironically, used to prevent miscarriage). By necessity, surrogates are also used when gay male couples desire children. Surrogates may use their own eggs (known as *traditional surrogacy*) or become impregnated with the intended parents' gametes or with some combination of eggs and/or sperm donors (known as *gestational surrogacy*). And, as in the use of donor technology, the surrogate can be known (a family member or friend) or can be someone who is solicited solely for the purpose of carrying the pregnancy.

Intended parents often worry about what it will be like for the surrogate to give up the baby after birth. It is typically believed that if a surrogate is not genetically tied to the baby she is carrying (i.e., a gestational surrogate), she will feel no attachment to it and have no difficulty relinquishing it to the intended parents. In most cases, this is true. It is testimony to the power of attachment, however, and the attachment of a woman to her unborn child, that surrogates can indeed become very attached to a baby in utero. They may suffer a genuine sense of loss when the baby is placed with the intended parents. This is not to say that a surrogate will not relinquish the baby—she is legally required to do so—but therapists must be prepared to help the surrogate work through her sense of loss and grieve both the pregnancy and the baby. Surrogates often feel ashamed of their grief, feeling that their altruism should somehow supercede any sense of loss; when they feel sad after the birth, they may feel selfish instead of generous, which can deal a blow to their sense of self. The clinician must also be attuned to postpartum depression or anxiety secondary to birth, which a surrogate herself may not be prepared for.

Surrogacy raises many moral, legal, and ethical issues, as well as psychological considerations. Although insurance companies often cover the medical costs associated with the pregnancy, couples who "rent a womb" may spend tens of thousands of dollars in remuneration. Because the legality of surrogacy in the United States varies from state to state, intended parents may need to "adopt" their baby from the surrogate mother; the legal line between where the birth mother's rights end and the intended parents' rights begin can be confusing. And because surrogacy is illegal in many countries, a new phenomenon, known as *medical tourism*, whereby people travel to other states or nations for their medical treatment, has been rapidly growing. Medical tourism for surrogacy is flourishing because of the legal restrictions in some countries but also because of the enormous costs involved. In India, for example, where surrogacy costs are a mere fraction of what it costs in the United States—$6,000 to $10,000 compared with upward of $80,000—surrogacy is estimated to be a $445-million-a-year industry (Warner, 2008).

Is it immoral or degrading for a woman to "sell" her body as a surrogate? As Warner (2008) pointed out, for poor Indian women, who can buy a house with the money they make as a surrogate, the answer is not necessarily clear. The sense of entitlement for couples with means may be off-putting, but, economically speaking, they may be helping more than hurting. Psychologically, however, as previously noted, carrying a pregnancy to term and then relinquishing that child (as in adoption) may be quite painful for some surrogates, even without any genetic ties. For some, as with the surrogates from India, the relationship may abruptly end after the baby is born. The intended mother may have mixed emotions about the surrogate: She may feel jealous of the surrogate for being able to carry her baby, and at the same time enormously indebted to her.

The reactions of other people may also be problematic for both the surrogate and the intended parents. Many people feel that a child born outside of the sanctity of marriage is immoral and see any third-party involvement as being unnatural or sacrilegious, especially if it involves a woman carrying a child that was not conceived with her husband. Some have gone so far as calling it adulterous. Additionally, as in donor technology, what to tell the child about his or her origins, and how the child may react, are all issues to consider. In working with couples contemplating surrogacy, or in consulting with surrogates, the mental health practitioner can help by bringing these concerns to the table and guiding all parties involved in this complex emotional process. The more informed each party is of the potential pitfalls and feelings they may have, the more likely that all will be satisfied with the outcome.

ADOPTION

Children who have been orphaned or relinquished by their biological parents have been adopted by other adults and incorporated into nonbiological families since antiquity. Adoption serves multiple purposes: It ensures the safety and development of children who need parents while, at the same time, it offers infertile couples the opportunity to become parents. There is a vast literature on adoption, far beyond the scope of this chapter to cover. Therefore, this section focuses on the emotional struggles infertile couples may face when making the decision to adopt, and, once the decision is made, the myriad options open to them.

Most couples who decide to adopt have been through the long and painful route of dealing with infertility. It has been estimated that 81% of couples who adopt children have not been able to have a biological child of their own (Ivaldi, 2000) and may view adoption as their last resort. In a study of infertile couples' experience with adoption, Daniluk and Hurtig-Mitchell (2003) found that couples saw adoption as a "backup plan" and something to consider when all else had failed. Although knowing that adoption was a possibility may have provided some comfort in getting through the trials of infertility, it was clearly not their first choice and required a shift in their thinking. From clinical observation, couples who view adoption as a choice, rather than feel resigned to it, are able to traverse this new roller coaster ride with more ease than those who feel forced into it.

Although third-party reproduction may be the right solution for some couples, for others it is not. Some may be tired of the medical and emotional demands of using assisted reproductive technology (ART), others may have ethical or religious views that prohibit its use, whereas others may prefer adoption because it is more socially sanctioned. Many couples feel that helping a child who already exists is preferable to "fooling with nature." Others weigh their financial constraints, comparing the low odds of having a child with ART with the virtual guarantee of an adopted child—if they can persevere through the equally arduous process of adoption. Whatever the reason, couples must grapple with the change in their reproductive story. The reconfiguration of the family to include a nonbiological child is not easy and may have multi-generational implications; it is a choice that needs to be carefully considered. Most important, the loss of a shared biological connection with the child needs to be grieved, along with the personal sense of inadequacy a couple may face in not being able to do what "everyone else can." It behooves the couple to recognize not only their own multiple losses but also the significant losses of the birth parents and the adoptee (Cudmore, 2005).

Many couples are fearful about the adoption process and the assessment they must go through. They feel scrutinized by the home study and judged by the birth parents. The evaluation process may feel unfair; after all, no one who is a biological parent must go through this kind of scrupulous appraisal. Couples may worry that they will be found unsuitable—wondering whether their house is too small, they make enough money, or they are too old. They may feel as if they have to sell themselves as being "good enough" and feel devastated if they are not chosen quickly. Once again couples may feel a loss of privacy and powerlessness, as their eligibility for parenthood is assessed and their future is yet again in the hands of others, this time not of physicians but of agencies, social workers, lawyers, and/or the birth parents (Cudmore, 2005; Daniluk & Hurtig-Mitchell, 2003). By labeling and validating these fears and worries, the mental health professional can reassure preadoptive parents that their feelings are normal and typical, which can help decrease some of this anxiety.

Couples may also worry that they will not love an adopted child as much as they would a biological one (Salzer, 2000). Likewise, they may have concerns that their extended family will not treat their adopted child as a "legitimate" family member (Daniluk & Hurtig-Mitchell, 2003). Indeed, there may be some who fear that family members will be unable to accept the child into the family as they would a biological offspring, especially if the child is of a different race or culture. The clinician can dispel these concerns, however, by again helping couples understand how attachment works. As discussed previously, attachment has more to do with the daily care and nurturance of a child—changing diapers, feeding, cultivating their development, and loving them—than with DNA. The more that adoptive parents feel this bond with their child, the less vulnerable they will feel to the opinions of others.

Inevitably, with adoption, the issue of nature versus nurture arises, with fears about the birth parent's lifestyle and background, and concerns about the child's prenatal environment. Questions abound—from conjecturing about the genetic determinants that will affect the child's personality to concerns about the birth mother's behavior during the pregnancy—did she smoke, take medication, abuse substances, eat too much junk food? This can create a terrible bind for prospective parents, as they must assess their own personal biases, prejudices, and limits as to what is acceptable to them. After trying for so long and hard to have a biological child, they may have doubts about someone who could relinquish a child. Having a greater understanding of the birth mother or birth family's circumstances will likely increase the adoptive parents' empathy, knowing that the decision to relinquish comes at great cost.

When chosen by a birth parent, adoptive parents may feel frightened to say no, afraid that they will have to wait months or even years before another offer comes their way. What if this is their only chance at parenthood? And what if the birth parents change their mind? After so much uncertainty and loss in dealing with infertility, the thought that they may lose their long-awaited child can be unbearable. For some, this can feel like such a threat that they choose international adoption instead of domestic, where there is no contact with the birth parents. The whole idea of "open adoption" may feel very risky to couples: The amount of contact that is negotiated may feel uncomfortable to the adoptive parents and may make them feel as if their relationship with their adoptive child is at risk. It is not uncommon for adoptive parents to fear that their child will reject them in preference to his or her birth parents. Again, the therapist, through a psychoeducational approach to treatment, can allay these fears. The therapist can explain, for example, that although there are certainly times when a birth mother will change her mind or an adopted child will prefer a relationship with the birth parents over the adoptive parents, these are the exceptions, not the norm. Nevertheless, especially right after the birth, adoptive parents may need to be encouraged to be self-protective, to recognize that they will not be without risk until after the adoption is final. This may entail not allowing themselves to become completely attached until the documents are signed—a difficult task when their whole being is aching to love that baby completely and consider it their own.

CHOOSING TO REMAIN CHILD-FREE

Perhaps the biggest shift in the reproductive story is to take the path that does not include parenting. After years of pursuing parenthood, clients who choose this path undoubtedly have endured significant losses in their self-esteem, relationships with their partners, and/or relationships with family and friends. Because social standards generally point to marriage and childrearing, childlessness is often considered an aberration (Campbell, 1986). Making the voluntary decision not to have children is difficult enough—it requires challenging the norm and societal expectations. When childlessness is involuntary, however, the intensity of feelings is significant and has been associated with substantial psychological distress (McQuillan, Greil, White, & Jacob, 2003). Involuntary childlessness requires a change in direction and a major restructuring of one's life, identity, and vision of the future.

As discussed earlier (see Chapter 2), the adult developmental milestones—separation/individuation, intimacy needs, identity issues, generativity—can be activated and readily achieved by the transition to parenthood. Does childlessness, then, imply developmental arrest and inability to attain adulthood? Absolutely not. Although becoming a parent provides a built-in structure, many possible routes exist to reach these developmental goals. Factors have been identified that help couples successfully adapt: high levels of support, marital and sexual satisfaction, good self-esteem, the development of an identity other than that of parent, the ability to nurture others, and meaningful pursuits in other areas of life (Daniluk & Tench, 2007; Rubin, 2002).

It can be very helpful in therapy to identify these factors as goals, as therapists guide patients into new avenues in their life. Patients who take action and problem solve seem to cope better with the end of their reproductive pursuit of biological parenting (Daniluk & Tench, 2007). It is not uncommon for patients to pursue a new career or hobby, return to school, volunteer for an organization that brings personal satisfaction—these are all areas in which couples can put their energy and gain a sense of control and fulfillment (Daniluk, 2001). Often, these activities include interacting with children or students. One man left his long-term career as a medical researcher to teach high school biology; a woman chose to volunteer at a center for homeless families; yet another assisted at an animal shelter with bottle-feeding abandoned kittens and puppies. Other couples may choose to embrace the freedom of childlessness to travel and explore the world. Whatever the activity, couples can rewrite their reproductive story to find happiness and meaning in roles other than parenthood.

It is vital for the patient, as well as the therapist, to recognize that this process—shifting from the long and arduous pursuit of becoming a parent to constructing an alternative lifestyle—can take a long time. It creates yet another identity crisis for people whose identity and sense of self has been under attack for years. It is a complicated decision, and most couples who decide to remain a family of two are hit with moments of doubt and pain. Couples should be made aware that even when they have made a thoroughly considered decision not to have children, they will continue to mourn, especially when life events reawaken their longing, such as when friends' children graduate or siblings or peers become grandparents. This does not mean that they made a wrong or bad decision, but rather this mourning should be normalized as part of the grieving process, which may last—with fading intensity—over the course of their lifetime.

SUMMARY

As individuals and couples deal with the multiple, complex, and emotionally laden choices available to them to create a family, it is normal for one solution to feel viable at one moment and impossible the very next. Each shift in the reproductive story—anywhere along the line from using oral medication to enhance fertility, to using injectables, IVF, donor technology, or adoption or the decision to remain a family of two—involves a loss that must be grieved. Because the list of possibilities and the wide-ranging emotions evoked can be overwhelming, the clinician can play an integral role in helping clients normalize their confusion and frustration. Allowing patients to try on new possibilities, while grieving the old, is essential in making decisions about their future reproductive story.

III
THERAPIST'S CONSIDERATIONS

8

SELF-DISCLOSURE, TRANSFERENCE, AND COUNTERTRANSFERENCE

The work of psychotherapy rests on the reality of the intensely personal relationship between patient and therapist, across theoretical orientations. Despite all efforts to remain neutral and objective, it is the nature of human interaction that verbal communication occurs against a backdrop of nonverbal cues, physical setting, personality, and cognitive style of both patient and therapist. Because of the intimacy of the therapeutic environment, it is inevitable that patients will have feelings and reactions to their therapist, and vice versa. This occurs both in a real sense, in the development of the working alliance, and in the unconscious realm, through the experience of transference and countertransference. Invariably, patients, who are all-revealing, will be curious about their therapists, who are, by nature of the relationship, much less so. In addition to the experience of transference and countertransference, the question of self-disclosure is important to address, especially when treating the unique needs of the reproductive patient. In this chapter, we discuss various theoretical viewpoints of therapist self-disclosure, with the aim of underscoring the technical challenges of working with this population.

Although it is hardly a prerequisite, it is not uncommon for therapists to become involved in reproductive psychology because of their own losses and trauma in trying to become a parent. Patients often ask, "What got you into this field?" or "Do you have any children?" These questions can be disarming for the clinician: Whether the therapist has children—or whether the therapist has gone through a reproductive trauma. How a therapist answers these questions—if, when, and how much to disclose—is highly personal and should be decided on a case-by-case basis. As we discuss later, although the decision may be influenced by the therapist's training and orientation, reproductive patients require some special considerations that at times run counter to traditional viewpoints. Regardless of theoretical perspective, however, self-disclosure must be done judiciously, ethically, and with extreme care.

Although for some clinicians their own reproductive trauma may be a thing of the past, others may experience a pregnancy loss during the course of psychotherapy or may be in the process of trying to conceive at the same time as the patient. In these particular circumstances, as illustrated later, special attention must be paid to the therapist–patient relationship and possible transference and countertransference reactions. Additionally, not all mental health practitioners have experienced reproductive problems; their reproductive stories may have proceeded without any trauma. Disclosure in this condition will likely create other transference feelings that need to be addressed in the therapy as well.

Working with infertility and reproductive loss clients can be extremely satisfying as they heal and as they rewrite and resolve their reproductive stories. On the other hand, the need to tolerate the multiple losses and traumas that patients suffer can take its toll on the therapist. Helping clients through a miscarriage, stillbirth, or perinatal death, or helping them decide to terminate a Down syndrome child, or supporting them during failed after failed cycles can be emotionally stressful for a therapist. It is hard to sit with patients who endure so much loss, to deal with death when one should be celebrating life. This chapter examines the risks and benefits of working with patients as they process their trauma and discusses ways in which the therapist can effectively cope with his or her own parallel or vicarious grief.

TO SELF-DISCLOSE OR NOT: THEORETICAL PERSPECTIVES

To fully understand the special needs and technical considerations when working with reproductive patients, it is helpful to be aware of the theoretical viewpoints on therapist self-disclosure in the general psychotherapy population. Much has changed in psychotherapy since Freud first discussed self-disclosure, suggesting that the therapist be "like a mirror" and reflect back only what the patient reveals (Freud, 1912/2000, p. 18). Traditional psychoanalytic theorists view self-disclosure as a detriment to the therapy process because it shifts the focus off of the patient and onto the therapist and can distort the patient's fantasies and transference by introducing "real" elements of the psychotherapist. More recent psychoanalytic–psychodynamic thinking posits not only that strict neutrality is impossible to maintain but also that revealing an authentic self may actually enhance the therapeutic experience (Bloomgarden & Mennuti, 2009; Knox & Hill, 2003). Even if a therapist never verbally reveals personal information, patients learn a great deal by observing the therapist's ethnicity, gender, style of office, and dress (Peterson, 2002; Stricker, 2003). Bloomgarden and Mennuti (2009) broadly defined *self-disclosure* as "anything that is revealed about a therapist verbally, nonverbally, on purpose, by accident, wittingly, or unwittingly, inclusive of information discovered about them from another source" (p. 8). Nonetheless, there is a distinction between the conscious, verbal communication that reveals information about the therapist and the unconscious or nonverbal cues that patients pick up on (Geller, 2003). Intentional and deliberate sharing of personal information is what most therapists identify as self-disclosure (Zur, 2009).

Other theoretical positions consider self-disclosure to be an integral part of therapy. Humanistic therapists, for example, feel that self-disclosure promotes genuineness in the therapist–client relationship (Rogers, 1951) and, as a result, helps clients to be more candid and disclose more of themselves. The clinician thus becomes a role model endorsing authenticity and trust (Lane & Hull, 1990). The therapist's openness validates and normalizes the client's plight and helps to minimize the power differential in the therapeutic relationship (Jourard, 1971). Similarly, those who practice from a feminist orientation believe that self-disclosure is a critical component of therapy. They advocate that appropriate disclosure helps to equalize power in the therapeutic relationship, reduces the patient's shame, and empowers the patient to make changes (Mahalik, VanOrmer, & Simi, 2000). Feminist therapists also feel that knowledge of the therapist's background and orientation is essential for the patient to give full informed consent (Peterson, 2002) because part of the philosophy of the therapy is to transmit feminist values to clients (Mahalik et al., 2000). Cognitive- or behaviorally oriented therapists believe that self-disclosure can challenge irrational thinking by providing feedback, normalizing problems, and modeling corrective behavior (Goldfried, Burckell, & Eubanks-Carter, 2003). Relational–cultural therapy focuses on mutual empathy and the therapeutic connection as the key to healing (Jordan, 2000). As such, a therapist's authentic reaction to the clients' suffering validates the client's experience and allows for a shared healing process to take place (Comstock, 2009).

Regardless of theoretical orientation, all therapists should keep several questions in mind when it comes to disclosure: Why is it important for the patient to know the information? How will the information affect the patient? Will it be helpful or harmful? What is the therapist's motivation to disclose? Is it truly to benefit the patient, or does it derive from the therapist's own needs? What should or should not be said? The most important issue always is "Is it in the patient's best interests?" The American Psychological Association (APA) has several guidelines for psychologists, which are related to the issue of self-disclosure (APA, 2002); the National Association for Social Workers (1999) and the American Counseling Association (2005) also have guidelines for licensed social workers and counselors, respectively. APA Ethical Principle A states, "Psychologists strive to benefit those with whom they work and take care to do no harm" (APA, 2002, p. 3). A good rule of thumb for all mental health practitioners, regardless of training, is to practice *nonmaleficence* (i.e., avoid doing harm to the patient) and *beneficence* (i.e., do what is helpful for the patient; Peterson, 2002). This code of conduct is echoed in APA Ethical Standards 3.04 (Avoiding Harm) and 3.08 (Exploitative Relationships). These standards recognize the power differential in the therapist–client relationship. Although the APA Ethics Code does not specifically discuss self-disclosure, "concerns about client exploitation often are raised in relation to therapist self-disclosure" (Peterson, 2002, p. 22). If the therapist is disclosing for his or her own needs, then disclosure clearly should not be part of the therapy and can be considered to be unethical. Using disclosure as a therapeutic tool can be quite valuable with some patients, particularly with reproductive patients, but with others it may actually hinder progress; thus, each case should be assessed, using sound clinical and thoughtful judgment.

So, under what circumstances should a therapist disclose, and what information is appropriate when working with the psychotherapy population in general and the reproductive population in particular? Research indicates that one of the most important considerations in therapist self-disclosure is for it to serve the client and the therapy (Knox & Hill, 2003). How a client may perceive the disclosure is "dependent on context and the place in time in the evolution of the therapeutic relationship" (Cornell, 2007, p. 54). If the therapeutic alliance is robust and positive, then the chances are that the disclosure will be received in a constructive manner. Myers and Hayes (2006) found that when the therapeutic relationship was sound, therapists received higher ratings if they made general disclosures (compared with no disclosures), but if the alliance was weak, the therapist's disclosures were perceived negatively. Thus, before any type of verbal self-disclosure is made, the mental health practitioner must be very aware of and attuned to the patient's history and needs (Goldstein, 1994). Other important factors to consider in self-disclosure are the client's age, culture, socioeconomic status, presenting problem, and diagnosis (Zur, 2009). The setting of the therapy is also significant; small towns or rural areas, for example, where one may run into clients in various community settings, may make disclosure unavoidable (Zur, 2009).

The content of a disclosure should also be approached considering the client's, not the therapist's, needs. It can be as benign as informing the patient of one's education and areas of specialty, or it can be something that is more personal in nature. Seven different types of therapist self-disclosures have been identified: those dealing with (a) *facts* (disclosing one's credentials and professional experience), (b) *feelings* (comparing one's own feelings in situations comparable to what the patient is describing), (c) *insight* (sharing perceptions of one's own life as similar to the patient's), (d) *strategy* (discussing how the therapist would handle a like circumstance), (e) *reassurance* or *support* (normalizing the patient's feelings by revealing one's own), (f) *challenge* (divulging personal experience that is the same as the patient's), and (g) *immediacy* (relating the patient's behavior with others to analogous behaviors the patient displays with the therapist; Knox & Hill, 2003). Clinicians may choose to disclose in order to model behavior or emotional expression, normalize clients' reactions, provide empathy and reassurance, and increase the sense of similarity between the therapist and the client (Peterson, 2002). These are particularly helpful justifications for self-disclosure when working with reproductive patients, once self-disclosure has been deemed appropriate. Equalizing the power in the therapeutic relationship (Jourard, 1971) and making the therapist seem more humane (Lane & Hull, 1990) also have been noted as factors that are beneficial to clients. "Clients' perception of therapists as more real and human . . . improved the therapy relationship and helped clients feel normal and reassured. Improvement in the therapy relationship, as well as feelings of normality and reassurance, then made clients feel better and enhanced their openness and honesty in therapy" (Knox & Hill, 2003, p. 532).

The amount of disclosure can affect the therapeutic relationship as well. Patients' perceptions of the clinician can vary, depending on how much is disclosed. In one of the few treatment outcome studies on therapist self-disclosure, Barrett and Berman (2001) found that an increased level of disclosure had the effect of decreasing symptoms. Additionally, patients liked their therapists more when disclosure was increased (Barrett & Berman, 2001). Although patients may perceive a therapist who never discloses as cold or distant, too much disclosure can be overwhelming to the patient. Patients may be confused or burdened by too much disclosure, feeling distracted from their own therapeutic needs. As we discuss further, this is especially important to remember when working with reproductive patients. Researchers' conclusions suggest that disclosure can be an effective treatment tool, but it should be used judiciously and only when it can promote therapeutic goals (Barrett & Berman, 2001; Hill & Knox, 2001; Knox & Hill, 2003; Peterson, 2002; Stricker, 2003).

DISCLOSURE TO REPRODUCTIVE PATIENTS

It is important for mental health practitioners to consider that working with this population is not the same as conducting psychotherapy with other kinds of patients. Patients with infertility and/or pregnancy loss do not enter therapy to make fundamental changes to their personality. Instead, they come to restore their sense of self, to grieve, and to get back to feeling whole again (Leon, 1996). With that in mind, clinicians may be called on to be more interactive and open in their approach. Although this may promote a different dynamic between therapist and patient, the therapist, as in all clinical situations, must always be aware that what he or she reveals—or not—can have an impact on the therapeutic alliance and the course of treatment.

With children at the forefront of their attention, it is not unusual for patients with reproductive concerns to wonder about their therapist's parental status. They may ask directly: Do you have any children? Or they may hint around: Why do you specialize in this area? Although these questions may appear to be benign and straightforward, it is imperative to recognize that, in fact, they are invariably emotionally loaded for the patient. These are extremely vulnerable patients, grief stricken and traumatized, who may suffer deep narcissistic wounds; questions about the therapist's reproductive circumstance can have many levels of meaning. They may be wondering whether the therapist is friend or foe, can understand them, or is like all the well-intentioned but misguided people who are insensitive to their needs. Hence how the therapist answers these types of questions depends not only on his or her orientation but also on the meaning of the question for each patient. When at all possible, it is important to explore why the question is being asked, before answering it directly. A psychoeducational statement about why the therapist wants to discuss the patient's feelings before answering the question may be helpful in order to avoid seeming distant or secretive.

Nancy, for example, is a new mother experiencing postpartum depression. Her reactions were complicated by the fact that, as a young child, she had witnessed her own mother's multiple miscarriages, including graphic details, as well as her mother's subsequent depression. When she wondered if the therapist had children, the therapist chose to explore Nancy's fantasies before answering the question. "I am happy to answer your question, Nancy," said the therapist. "But sometimes people have reactions to the therapist's personal story that can distract them from their own experience. Before I answer, let's talk about what you think about when you wonder if I have children." This proved to be very useful. Nancy admitted that she always pictured her therapist as a kind of "earth mother," living out in the country, "barefoot and pregnant" with lots of babies. This image seemed to serve as a counterpoint to her frightening memories of her own mother's reproductive failures. Mildly disparaging of the therapist, it also revealed the unconscious competitiveness that had made it difficult for Nancy to feel close to women. Of great significance, it became the catalyst for Nancy's acknowledgment of her sense of guilt that she had conceived easily when her mother had suffered. It was this guilt that in part fueled her postpartum depression. Through her depression, Nancy was able to suffer like her mother did; not allowing herself to enjoy her baby became her punishment for her competitiveness with her mother. Interestingly, after sharing and examining these fantasies, the patient retracted her question, noting that she preferred to maintain the fantasy rather than deal with her reactions to the truth. This is not uncommon and tends to occur when the patient believes that the answer will cause anxiety rather than relief. If, after some discussion, or at least after being offered the opportunity to talk about it, a patient still wants to know, then the therapist can decide how to answer.

Reproductive patients will have feelings and reactions not just about whether the therapist has children but also about the therapist's actual reproductive story. Some patients may feel relieved, for example, to know the therapist has gone through similar losses. Many patients experience an enormous amount of shame in their fertility status, almost as if they were pariahs in a child-centered universe. If a therapist reveals that he or she also struggled to have a child, or had a pregnancy loss, or a premature birth, patients may breathe a sigh of relief: Here is someone who understands and is human, who they can truly identify with. This serves to decrease the patient's feelings of shame and equalizes the power differential between patient and therapist (Jourard, 1971; Knox, Hess, Peterson, & Hill, 1997; Peterson, 2002). Patients may also feel hopeful and see the therapist as a role model; if the therapist has survived his or her own trauma, there is a good possibility that the patient will, too.

If clients know about their therapist's reproductive loss, however, they may worry that their story will become a burden to the therapist. They may feel the need to take care of the therapist by minimizing their own grief and loss in order to protect the therapist. Miriam Greenspan, a feminist therapist, openly discussed the loss of her infant son with her clients. She noted that "a sudden dose of reality hit hard and became a part of the therapeutic process" (Greenspan, as cited in Comstock, 2009, p. 263). Greenspan discussed her reproductive trauma as breaking through her clients' fantasies that she was all-powerful. Rather than deny what had happened, she utilized it in the treatment process. "It didn't interfere with the work. If they were feeling bad for me or wanted to protect me, they would tell me, and we would work on that" (Greenspan, as cited in Comstock, 2009, p. 264).

One of the risks clinicians take in disclosing their own experience to the reproductive patient is that, rather than feeling relieved or more connected, the patient may feel a sense of alienation or competition with the therapist. For example, a successful outcome to the therapist's reproductive struggles can give the patient hope, but, conversely, an unsuccessful outcome can add to the patient's despair. If this is addressed, the clinician can use the material as a therapeutic opportunity and explore the patient's reactions to the therapist's self-disclosure. Asking how they feel about what was revealed can be essential to the ongoing psychological dialogue and treatment (Knox & Hill, 2003). If the reaction remains unaddressed, it can create an unconscious rift between them, as the following example illustrates.

Kathy, a 35-year-old editor, had been trying to conceive for 5 years. She sought supportive therapy prior to her third in vitro fertilization (IVF) procedure. Kathy felt the therapy to be very helpful and liked the therapist, but a whole year passed before she asked about the therapist's reproductive story. At first, she only asked if the therapist had been through infertility (she had) and only after discussing this did she ask whether the therapist had been successful in having children (she had). On the surface, Kathy appeared happy for the therapist and hopeful for herself; she expressed feeling reassured to know that people do come through these traumas intact.

A week later, however, Kathy reported a dream: "I was at work, and there was a tall fence in the yard. I was on one side and everybody else was on the other, and I could not get through the fence. I felt so alone—and angry. I did not understand why I wasn't allowed to be the same as everybody else." Kathy interpreted this dream as consciously pertaining to her isolation and jealousy of friends and colleagues who were having babies, about feeling different and set apart from them. When the therapist wondered if the dream also related to Kathy's learning about the therapist's reproductive history the previous week, Kathy became defensive. "Oh, no," she exclaimed. "I would never feel angry at you about that. I appreciated your being honest, and I felt happy for you. What kind of person would I be if I didn't?"

As the therapist gently explored this, Kathy acknowledged how guilty she often felt about her jealousy of her pregnant friends. Feeling envious added to the self-criticism she already felt for being unable to conceive. The therapist was aware that, unconsciously, Kathy's dream was almost certainly a reference to an unspoken rift between them—with her and her children on one side of the fence and Kathy, childless, on the other. But it was also clear to the therapist that, at this point in the therapy, and in her reproductive story, Kathy was unable to tolerate any negative feelings toward the therapist; her need to feel connected and close to the therapist served as an important antidote to the loneliness she felt in her social world, and the therapist chose not to confront the denial. Nevertheless, although Kathy needed to deny her transference reactions, bringing up the possibility of such feelings did help her recognize and normalize her internal conflicts about her friends, which in itself provided some relief. These are feelings that patients face on a daily basis in their lives, with friends and family having children all around them; it can be enormously therapeutic to discharge these negative feelings in a safe place and to develop strategies, with the therapist as an ally, to cope with the "outside world."

One of the issues regarding therapist self-disclosure to reproductive patients is whether the therapist's struggle has been resolved or not. It may happen that the therapist is trying to conceive at the same time as the patient or has experienced a reproductive loss during the therapy. The therapist may be distracted by his or her own traumatic experiences or may be pulled away from regular clinical hours for tests and monitoring. If clinicians disclose their unresolved struggles, they may not be able to be sufficiently objective. Although this situation may enhance the therapist's empathy for the patient's circumstances, it may also increase the risk of boundary violations. The therapist should take extra caution in these circumstances not to use the therapy for his or her own needs. One suggestion is for the therapist not to disclose any issues that do not have sufficient resolution (Knox & Hill, 2003).

There may be times, however, when disclosure of the therapist's loss is impossible to keep private. Dana Comstock (2009) wrote about the complications midway through her first pregnancy, resulting in the premature and stillbirth of her daughter. The medical emergency that she experienced, followed by a 3-month absence, necessitated telling her students and clients. When she did return to her work, she was able to use her loss constructively with her clients. Keeping the focus on her client's needs, she stated, "Our work shifted to a deeper level as my loss had created an opportunity for them to also explore how life can turn on a dime" (Comstock, 2009, p. 263). She also noted that extensive details of the clinician's experience do not need to be discussed. Simply saying, "I, too, have lost a baby" or "although my circumstances are different from yours, I, too, have experienced a reproductive trauma" can instill a sense of trust and understanding.

If the therapist is struggling with his or her own reproductive issues, clinical work may provide a sense of relief. Focusing on the patient's needs rather than on one's own may allow the therapist to gain some distance from his or her personal strife (Freeman, 2005). On the other hand, because of the intensity of emotions during infertility treatment or pregnancy loss, clinicians may have difficulty, when asked about their personal life, in being open and authentic about their own experience. They may feel a deep sense of shame, just as patients do. Therapists do have a right to privacy and may not be comfortable exposing themselves. The clinician must be sensitive, however, to the patient's vulnerability and be extra tactful in explaining why he or she does not want to self-disclose.

If the therapist does not feel comfortable sharing information, for example, he or she could say something like, "It is completely normal that you want to know more about me, because you want to be sure I will understand you. But, for my own personal reasons, I would rather not discuss this right now. It has nothing to do with you, so please do not take it personally; it is just something I would rather put on the back burner for the moment." Although most patients will accept this, others may react negatively or even choose to see another therapist. Patients can easily feel rebuffed or criticized by the therapist's need for privacy, which can then increase their own sense of shame. As with almost all aspects of work with reproductive patients, there is no formula for handling these situations. Therapists must try to stay in tune with their own emotions, so that they can respond sensitively to the patient's. The following is an example of how one clinician handled it.

Yvonne was in therapy throughout her infertility treatment. She often spoke glowingly of her physician, who was a renowned specialist. After much consideration, her therapist, who was undergoing infertility treatment with a different doctor, decided to switch to this specialist as well. The therapist was very nervous that she would run into Yvonne in the waiting room, yet she also wanted the best medical care for herself. After experiencing increasing anxiety, the therapist chose to tell Yvonne directly that she, too, was a patient of this doctor. They agreed that, if they ever saw each other at the doctor's office, they would greet each other politely, but maintain distance. Because Yvonne was apprised of the situation and included in a discussion of how to cope with it, she felt both closer to the therapist and also more understanding and respectful of her therapist's needs. Furthermore, if a question ever came up about the therapist's medical treatment, she made a point of underlining that she and Yvonne had different needs and that one treatment "did not fit all," thereby skirting the risk of comparison and judgment.

What happens if one or the other conceives during the therapy? As in the present example, with both the patient and therapist in fertility treatment at the same time, there is a good chance that one or the other will become pregnant. Should the therapist become pregnant, self-disclosure eventually becomes a necessity. How to let patients know, when to tell them, and how to deal with their reactions are not easy questions. One possibility is for the therapist to caution the patient up front about her potential reactions, allowing the patient to be prepared to process the news rather than being stunned by it. The therapist may say something to the effect of, "I have always been honest with you, and something has come up that you will have many feelings about. It is important that we talk about them and then decide how to proceed. As you may or may not know, I have been undergoing infertility treatment. Like yours, it has been a grueling process. I have recently learned that I am pregnant . . . ." On the other hand, the clinician may not want to reveal anything about the pregnancy early on but may want to wait until the physical signs are apparent. Although this makes perfect sense from the therapist's perspective and honors her right to privacy, the patient also has rights, and he or she may choose to discontinue the therapeutic relationship because of the pregnancy. With news of the clinician's pregnancy, the client may feel inhibited to express anger or resentment and may have fantasies about being abandoned. Because patients may have a wide range of feelings—they may feel deceived, betrayed, envious, or hurt—the therapist must be acutely aware of the patient's needs.

Although challenging for both client and therapist, there are ways in which this unique situation can actually enrich the therapeutic experience. One patient, Leslie, at first felt panicked when she heard of her therapist's pregnancy. She was worried that she would not be able to stand going through the therapist's pregnancy, when she herself was so despairing about her own infertility. But she also felt very close to her therapist and couldn't bear to think of not seeing her anymore. With the therapist's support, Leslie was able to articulate both her fondness and happiness for her therapist, as well as her envy and resentment. This turned out to be very helpful, as it gave her confidence in her ability to cope. Leslie found that she was less anxious when friends or coworkers became pregnant, now that she knew she could tolerate the feelings. It also gave her hope that she too might eventually become a parent. If clients can work through their anger at their therapist's pregnancy and deal with the grief that yet another person is pregnant and they are not, it is possible that this experience will serve them well. However, therapists should also be aware that the patient may not be able to tolerate these feelings and may drop out of therapy; it is important that the therapist not take this personally or view it as a treatment failure.

If the situation is reversed, if the client should get pregnant while the therapist is also trying to conceive, the therapist must reconcile his or her own feelings and not jeopardize the therapeutic alliance. If the patient knows the therapist is "trying," she may feel guilty about her own success or feel the need to take care of the therapist. The patient must be reassured that the therapist has her own network of support. Indeed, in this circumstance, it is recommended that the clinician seek outside consultation. In a parallel process to that of the patient, the therapist can also work through these painful issues and grow from the experience, just as Leslie did when her therapist became pregnant.

Although therapists who are in the midst of their own reproductive crises may have enormous understanding and empathy for their patients, awareness of the clinician's situation may not serve the best interests of the patient. The interpersonal dynamic may, in fact, feel like a burden to the patient. If a patient feels as if the therapy session is about the therapist's needs, or feels put in the role of taking care of the therapist, clearly something is amiss. As stated earlier, an essential rule of thumb for therapists to follow is to promote what is best for the patient (beneficence) and to do no harm (nonmaleficence;

Peterson, 2002), even if it means referring the patient to another clinician. Therapists, in the middle of their own emotionally difficult time, may be too vulnerable to be effective with a particular patient who brings up similar feelings and should refer the patient to someone else: "Because of my own circumstances, I don't feel that I can provide the kind of help and support you need right now. I think it would be best for you to work with someone else." Clinicians may, in fact, choose to postpone working with this population until they have gained some distance from their own trauma. The therapist must do enough of his or her own healing to be able to assist others with comparable experiences (Anonymous, 2007).

For those clinicians who have not had firsthand experience with a reproductive trauma and have had children easily, or for those clinicians who do not have children, dealing with this clientele presents other complications on the issue of disclosure. When patients feel that "so many people don't get it," they may worry that the therapist is yet another person who doesn't understand. Among the general psychotherapeutic population, therapists are often asked if they have gone through the specific problem that the client is coping with, be it addiction, depression, divorce, or any other emotional experience. Clearly, therapists do not have to experience every trauma that may befall humans to be good clinicians. If the practitioner who has not gone through a reproductive trauma chooses to disclose, he or she should do so truthfully and then reassure the patient of his or her clinical expertise and empathy.

It can be helpful to provide other examples of how therapists are effective, even if they have not had the same experiences as the patient; an excellent and obvious illustration is that therapists often treat patients of the opposite gender. The therapist can underline the two-person model of therapy (Hoffman, 1992; Ogden, 1994); that is, that even if the therapist has not experienced exactly the same thing as the patient, he or she is interested in understanding what it is like. Although one does not necessarily want to put the patient in the position of having to "teach" the therapist, in fact, being able to inform others about the experience of reproductive trauma is a skill that patients often wish they had. Patients often face well-intentioned but misguided friends, family members, or even strangers who are insensitive to their needs; therefore, knowing how to communicate these needs can be very helpful and such communication can be practiced in therapy. Furthermore, it is important for the therapist to encourage the patient to talk about misunderstandings that may arise in the therapeutic setting and to convey that the therapist can tolerate any negative reactions the patient may be having. This can be enormously helpful, especially if the patient is not able to confront friends or family when they don't "get it."

SUMMARY OF DISCLOSURE ISSUES

The issue of therapist self-disclosure is complex and has been much debated in the literature. The following summarizes some general questions clinicians should ask themselves regarding self-disclosure and addresses specific ways it might affect reproductive patients:

- Is the disclosure in the interest of the patient, or is it based on the needs of the therapist? If disclosure does not promote a therapeutic goal, then the clinician should not do so (Stricker, 2003). Disclosure to a reproductive patient that the therapist has experienced reproductive difficulties may enhance the therapeutic alliance, promote a sense of normalcy for the patient, and reduce shameful feelings. It may give patients a sense of hope that they, too, can get through this difficult time in their life. On the other hand, disclosure of the therapist's reproductive status may spark feelings of jealousy, competition, and isolation. Although this may feel burdensome to the patient, it could be of value, because the client can work out these negative feelings in the safety of the therapeutic setting.

- How much and how often should the mental health practitioner disclose? The general rule is to disclose infrequently and with care (Maroda, 2009). Sometimes the less said the better. Specifics of the therapist's life are less important than the patient's need to be understood. For example, the therapist can say, "My own reproductive story did not go as I had hoped either." Without going into details, the therapist has let the patient know that they, too, have suffered on their journey to create a family.

- What are the reasons for disclosure? It is not merely the content of the self-disclosure that is important, but it is also the reason *why* the therapist deems disclosure to be necessary that must be evaluated (Peterson, 2002). Again the interest of the patient should be kept in the forefront. In cases of infertility and/or pregnancy loss, therapist disclosure may help to build the therapeutic alliance, reduce the patient's feelings of shame and isolation, and validate and normalize negative emotions.

- Will disclosure influence the patient's own decisions? Therapists often serve as role models for their patients, and, in this sense, knowing how the therapist resolved his or her own reproductive crisis could be helpful. However, it is essential that therapists maintain neutrality as patients consider their options. It is not unusual for clients to mull over many solutions—and even change their minds any number of times. If the therapist is too invested in one preference over another (especially if this was the choice the therapist made), objectivity may be lost, and the patient may feel judged or criticized for whatever decision he or she makes.

- How should therapists respond if they are in the midst of their own struggles? Disclosure is much riskier if the therapist has not resolved his or her own issues (Knox & Hill, 2003), and it bears reiterating that the underlying ethical premise of self-disclosure must be a focus on the patient's needs and not the therapist's. If the therapist is going through an IVF cycle, for example, her own anxiety may interfere with clarity in helping the client with his or her reproductive struggles. The therapist may decide to refer a new client elsewhere, but, rather than not working with certain patients, it makes sense for the therapist to seek consultation with a supervisor or other therapist. If some disclosure is deemed necessary, a brief statement will suffice. Too much information may overwhelm the patient and turn the focus away from the patient's needs to the therapist's. The patient should never feel the need to take care of the therapist.

TRANSFERENCE AND COUNTERTRANSFERENCE ISSUES

The issue of self-disclosure is intrinsically tied to the concepts of transference and countertransference. Indeed, as we have discussed, decisions about self-disclosure must be made in the context of these dynamics. As in all therapeutic relationships, the feelings a reproductive patient has for his or her therapist, and vice versa, need to be in the forefront of the therapist's awareness. Whether unconsciously or verbalized, patients have transference reactions to their therapists and will wonder about their therapist: about his or her personal life, relationships, and—key for reproductive patients—whether he or she has children.

In turn, therapists have internal reactions to their patients. Consciously or not, subtly or overtly, therapists may feel pulled to treat various patients differently. As a therapist, one may have a "favorite" patient or, on the opposite end of the spectrum, one that is particularly difficult. These countertransference experiences can provide a useful guide to understanding the patient's dynamics. What's important to keep in mind is that therapists' feelings about patients may influence the ability to remain neutral.

A survey of Finnish infertility specialists described an "ideal" female infertility patient as healthy, in her early 30s, and with a good temperament and a lifestyle that is not centered on her career. They also favored women in stable, heterosexual relationships. In contrast, less appropriate patients were those with complicated health problems and psychosocial difficulties. These physicians were in a position to determine who would receive assisted reproductive technology, and so their perceptions of patients were critical (Malin, 2003). Mental health practitioners, especially those who screen patients for IVF, donor treatment, or adoption, may find themselves in a position similar to a gatekeeper. One study was conducted, for example, that examined attitudes of psychologists toward gay and lesbian parenting. Psychologists were given vignettes to rate, which were identical except for the sexual orientation of the adoptive parents and the gender of the child. Although most psychologists in the study were open-minded, the results did indicate that gay men and lesbians coupled with a female child were less likely to receive a recommendation for adoption than their heterosexual counterparts (Crawford, McLeod, Zamboni, & Jordan, 1999). These studies demonstrate the need to keep one's own personal biases out of an evaluation while using clinical judgment to determine "good" versus "bad" candidates.

What if the practitioner and patient differ in their beliefs regarding moral, ethical, or spiritual issues? For example, what if a woman decides to abort because of the gender of the child? What if the couple decides to remain child-free, but the therapist is invested in their having a baby? What if a couple continues to pursue the quest for a biological child when the likelihood of success is next to nothing? Is it the therapist's role to be a gatekeeper and make decisions about who should become a parent or not? What may be the right course for the patient may not be right for the therapist, and vice versa. The therapist must remain impartial and supportive and not try to influence the client but, rather, must guide the patient to arrive at his or her own reproductive decisions. This is especially important if the therapist is ambivalent or anxious about her own choices. For example, if the therapist is at the point of adopting, exhausted and depleted, she may not be able to tolerate it if her patient makes negative comments about adoption; she may, in fact, directly or indirectly encourage the patient to adopt as well, in part to justify her own decision. These kinds of situations make consultation with other mental health professionals crucial.

Although it is clearly not the therapist's role to make decisions for his or her clients, there are times when challenging their beliefs may be necessary. For example, one therapist, Dr. S., had a patient, Diane, who had endured 15 years of infertility, multiple surgeries, IVFs, losses, and traumas. Dr. S. had become very anxious about her patient's judgment and inability to stop treatment, yet she did not want to seem critical or nonsupportive. This dilemma was informed by the experience of a longtime friend of Dr. S., who had experienced 10 years of infertility and who had worked with a therapist throughout. Something her friend had said had stuck with Dr. S. for years: "I think I kept going because my doctor was so determined to get me pregnant. In retrospect, it makes me really angry that no one, not even my former therapist, confronted me and helped me to stop. Had I known how wonderful it would be to adopt, I never would've gone on for so long and put myself through so much."

This conversation had a deep impact on Dr. S. It led her to question whether her consistent neutrality toward her current patient was appropriate, but she worried that her patient would feel criticized or unsupported if she confronted her. Dr. S. finally chose to speak directly to the patient about her concerns. She decided that the risk of not confronting the patient's relentless pursuit of a medically impossible result was more damaging than the risk of talking about it; she ultimately felt that if the patient experienced her comments as critical, it was a reaction that could be discussed and worked through. "You know, Diane," she began, making a particular effort to be compassionate, "as I listen, I find myself in somewhat of a dilemma. In our work I have seen my role as someone who is neutral and accepting, as someone who is here to support you through this terribly traumatic experience of infertility. At the same time, I feel my job is to protect you from harm, and to help you see where there may be gaps in your understanding. I am reminded of someone I know who experienced years of traumatic infertility treatment and who was very angry that her therapist had never helped her to consider stopping. So I have to share with you some of my thoughts, and hope that you understand that they come from my deepest concern for your well-being. I know that you are extremely attached to your infertility doctor and that he is a marvelous physician. But it also seems that he is so invested in getting you pregnant that you have been unable to consider how unrealistic success is at this point. I am concerned that your judgment about your care has been clouded by your love for your doctor and your shared wish that you conceive. I am worried for your physical health and for your emotional exhaustion, and I would like to encourage you to think about what is keeping you from accepting this loss and moving towards another approach."

Diane's eyes filled with tears. Far from being defensive, she looked enormously relieved. "I have wanted to stop," she lamented. "But I can't seem to stop unless my doctor tells me definitively that I won't get pregnant, and because the cause has not been diagnosed, he cannot unequivocally say that."

"I can appreciate that," Dr. S. responded. "But there are many aspects of life in which we cannot have scientific proof, but the experiential proof informs our decisions. We know that there is a world under the surface of the sea, even though we can't directly see it. We know that there are stars in the sky, even if there are clouds and we can't visually prove their presence. I worry that you are unable to let yourself 'know' the reality of your situation, because you can't 'prove it' just as if you needed to deny that there are stars in the sky if you can't see them." Although Dr. S. felt somewhat anxious having this conversation, she knew that it was necessary, and Diane's sense of relief at "calling a spade a spade" was palpable. In fact, the patient went on to reassure the therapist that she had become aware of her doctor's overinvestment in her and that she did feel a need to at least determine an "exit plan," whereby, for example, she would agree to one more frozen cycle, but it would be clear to all that it would be the last one. She actually thanked Dr. S. for being forthright and clearly felt the therapist's concern for her. Of course, the circumstances behind such an intervention must be evaluated in a case-by-case manner, taking into account the complex psychosocial issues for each couple. But sometimes what is best for the patient is not served by blanket neutrality, and the therapist must be prepared to address this.

COPING WITH LOSS: THE THERAPIST'S PERSPECTIVE

The nature of working with clients in the throes of reproductive trauma necessitates dealing with a great deal of loss. Although it can be quite fulfilling to help clients traverse and heal from their reproductive traumas, it can have a negative effect on the therapist as well. One may rejoice with one's clients over a positive pregnancy test, but with a failed cycle or pregnancy demise, their devastation may become one's own. Over and over, therapists listen to tales of frustration, sadness, defeat, and death; these stories are painful and often hard to hear. For the therapist, knowing when to seek consultation and support for oneself is just as important as the clinical work.

Part of the healing process for patients is to be able to talk about the darkest parts of their story. These are the thoughts that haunt people in the middle of the night, causing them to relive the most frightening, and sometimes gruesome, aspects of their reproductive events. Clinical experience suggests that people often keep these thoughts to themselves because they are so awful; they fear that they will alienate or disgust the therapist if they reveal them. Patients may also be afraid they will be judged for the events; many find themselves replaying the details to assuage their guilt. As we have discussed, so many clients feel they did something wrong to cause their trauma and blame themselves: "What if I had called the doctor sooner? What if I had refused when they sent me home from the hospital?" Patients judge themselves—wrongly—for myriad possible explanations for their loss. The process of telling another person, who is "safe" and nonjudgmental, who can reassure them they are not to blame, is enormously therapeutic for clients.

Similarly, it can be beneficial for a patient who has had a stillbirth, for example, to bring in photographs of the baby and/or the baby's memory box, when he or she feels able. Patients are sometimes surprised if the therapist requests to see these mementos; they may be in disbelief that anyone else would want to share their grief. By viewing these keepsakes, the therapist is giving tacit acknowledgment that this was a real person, a real event. If the baby was named, the clinician should use this name when referring to the child. Again, this helps validate the patient's experience and gives him or her permission to talk about the child.

One of the most difficult experiences is when a patient must make a decision about the termination of a pregnancy. These poignant moments can be heartbreaking for patients and therapists alike. Clients who find themselves in this predicament may feel an added layer of guilt and shame in consciously making the choice to abort the pregnancy. These situations may bring up basic moral, ethical, and religious values, which the therapist may or may not share with the patient. Although the therapist may have certain ideas of what is right, these may be counter to the needs of the patient. Whatever the therapist's own personal stance, it is what is in the best interest of the patient that needs to be addressed. If the therapist adheres to a particular religious viewpoint, for instance, which prohibits abortion under any circumstance, it may be extremely difficult to support the patient. Even if the therapist does not have religious beliefs that conflict with those of the patient, different circumstances may make him or her uncomfortable. If a patient is considering terminating a pregnancy when it is not medically necessary, for example, a Down syndrome baby, or reducing multiples from two to one, the therapist must take note of his or her own feelings. If the therapist is the parent of multiples, or has a Down syndrome child himself, he may be anxious or critical about the patient's choice, especially if he is ambivalent about his own decision. The therapist will have to be extremely careful not to exhibit disapproval or judgment and keep the client's feelings central to the therapy. This is not to say that the various sides of an issue should not be discussed; it is vital for patients to thoroughly think through life-altering decisions. But, ultimately, it is the patient's choice. They must live with whatever decision they make.

Seeing disturbing photos, hearing upsetting details of loss, helping a couple through agonizing decisions—these activities can be emotionally draining for the therapist. Doing this therapy is not work for the faint of heart. There is a risk of the therapist being traumatized vicariously through the need to sit with the patient's pain. Sometimes, therapists are left with feelings of help-lessness as they watch their clients grieve. They may feel pulled to try "to fix" the problems; in the effort to take away the pain patients experience, therapists may overlook the value in their ability to "just listen." Clients need to tell their story and need to tell it many times; this is a significant part of the grieving process. With each telling, various details may be remembered and highlighted, and their experience can be understood in a different light. In a process parallel to what patients feel when they unburden themselves, therapists can profit from talking with others in the field. Seeking consultation allows clinicians to release their own anxiety over their patients' reproductive events.

If the therapist does not feel that he or she can truly be neutral and support the patient through whatever decision the patient makes, it is best for all concerned to refer the patient to another clinician. Often, therapists worry about making such a referral, fearing that the patient will feel rejected. One can convey the recommendation in a very supportive way, however. "This is truly one of the most painful and complex decisions you will ever face. As much as I care about you, I don't feel that I can provide the kind of guidance through this part of the process that you need. I have a colleague who specializes in this particular kind of trauma, and I would prefer that you consult with him/her; I feel I would be doing you a disservice to try to help you navigate this particular problem."

SUMMARY

Therapists are often drawn into the field of reproductive psychology because of their own difficulties in having children. This can prove to be a valuable resource; the therapist can tap into his or her own experiences to better empathize with patients. Whether to disclose one's own circumstances and how much to disclose should be addressed on a case-by-case basis and may greatly depend on one's theoretical stance. Whatever the theoretical orientation, however, disclosure should occur only if it will enhance the therapy and help the patient, not to serve the therapist's needs. In any case, hearing stories of multiple losses and psychological pain can be difficult, and therapists need to address their own feelings stirred up by the work. Seeking consultation is highly recommended for cases that are emotionally difficult, especially if they touch on the therapist's own reproductive loss.

9

ADJUNCTS TO THERAPY
AND COMPLEMENTARY CARE

The use of support groups for reproductive clients, either peer- or therapist-run, is a common addition to individual or couples psychotherapy. These groups, for infertility or pregnancy loss, can feel like lifesavers to patients, providing validation and a much-needed sense of belonging and understanding. Similarly, the Internet, which serves as a readily available research tool for medical and technical information, also provides access to others who are in a comparable plight. Clients can "chat," "blog," or "tweet" with other people at all times of the day and night, all across the world. Because of this anonymous connection, they may be able to open up in a way they cannot in face-to-face contact. Through monitored sites, they can also get answers from physicians or therapists—perhaps to questions they feel embarrassed to ask their own doctors.

Patients also routinely seek complementary care to their medical treatment, using Chinese herbs, acupuncture, yoga, massage therapy, diet, self-help books, or other mind–body techniques. In their effort to leave no stone unturned in the quest to have a baby, clients will try just about anything. Sometimes just knowing that they have tried everything—done it all "right"—provides relief. There can be downsides, however, to these adjuncts to treatment: People in support groups get pregnant, leaving others behind; as much as the Internet provides useful facts, there is also a great deal of misinformation; clients may be vulnerable to unproven "cures"; and patients can be overwhelmed by all the alternative treatments available to them. This chapter highlights both the positive and negative aspects of these additions to psychotherapy and counseling and illustrates, with clinical examples, the therapist's role as a neutral sounding board.

SUPPORT GROUPS

These days, support groups can be found for almost any medical or psychological condition. A review of therapy groups over the past 100 years has found them to be an effective means to help people through difficult periods in their life (Barlow, Burlingame, & Fuhriman, 2000). Studies of breast cancer patients, for example, who participated in short-term structured groups, were shown to have decreased anxiety and depression lasting 6 months postsessions (Hosaka, Tokuda, & Sugiyama, 2000) and enhanced survival rates (Spiegel, Bloom, Kraemer, & Gottheil, 1989). In terms of reproductive issues, groups can be found that deal with general infertility, specific diagnoses, or third-party reproduction matters. There are pregnancy loss groups and groups that deal with pregnancy termination, as well as groups that deal with the stresses of subsequent pregnancies and adoption. A simple search on the Internet can provide clients with information on groups all over the world. Groups may be gender specific or may be structured for couples, may be run by a peer who has experienced a similar life situation or by a trained medical or mental health professional, and may be run on a drop-in basis or have a specified number of sessions. For patients, seeking out others who have experienced similar life conditions provides hope, support, catharsis, and education (Daniels, 1993).

From a biopsychosocial perspective of infertility and pregnancy loss, the use of group interventions makes perfect sense. Research suggests that the psychological impact of infertility can be mediated in part by social support (Gerrity, 2001), but over the often-long course of medical treatment, patients often experience a decline in the traditional arenas of support from family and friends. Indeed, one of the most devastating effects of reproductive traumas is the sense of isolation that patients feel. As previously discussed, clients complain that they no longer fit in with peers who are either pregnant or who have babies. Their social world may shrink as more and more members of their cohort move on in their lives, whereas patients feel as if they are standing still. This is especially true if clients are dealing with primary infertility or the loss of first pregnancy. It bears repeating that although their *psychological* framework may have shifted into parenthood, their lack of a child keeps them feeling disconnected from others who have children. They may they feel awkward not only with friends or family who *do* have children but also with those who *don't*. They may no longer share the same interests or focus with their friends who are not yet ready to start a family. They may feel stuck in an in-between, socially "nowhere" state, in which the understanding they seek is not readily apparent. Finding a group of people who have undergone a similar reproductive trauma seems to help clients realize they are not alone, allows them to find like-minded friends, and offers them a place to share their pain, anger, and grief (Menning, 1976).

The literature on groups for infertile couples points to two different formats: Those that are emotionally based versus those that are problem-focused or cognitive–behavioral in orientation. *Emotionally based* groups are geared primarily toward regulating negative affect about the stressful event, whereas *problem-focused* groups are directed at controlling or modifying the problem (Lazarus & Folkman, 1984). Because reproductive traumas encompass the need for both emotional regulation (release of feelings, need for support, validation) and problem-solving strategies (need for information regarding diagnosis and treatment options, communication with medical personnel), both types of interventions have been found to be useful (McQueeney, Stanton, & Sigmon, 1997). In their study of infertile women, McQueeney et al. (1997) compared pre-, post-, and 1-month follow-up scores of an emotion-focused, problem-focused, and control group; they found that both intervention groups were significantly less distressed than the control group at the end of treatment.

Other studies have also demonstrated that group interventions can be helpful in dealing with many different aspects of reproductive crises for both men and women. One such study examined the efficacy of cognitive–behavioral groups for couples during the process of in vitro fertilization (IVF) treatment (McNaughton-Cassill, Bostwick, Arthur, Robinson, & Neal, 2002). Results showed that women who attended group sessions had a significant reduction in anxiety and depression upon completion of psychological treatment. Although men did not show a difference in levels of anxiety or depression, those who participated in the groups were more optimistic on posttreatment measures than those who were in a waiting-list control group. In an extensive review of the literature on psychosocial interventions in infertility, Boivin (2003) found that men and women both benefited, but in different ways. Men liked the practical information and advice they received from support groups, whereas women profited from the validation of their feelings from others and the sense of belonging (Boivin, 2003). Additionally, group interventions were found to be helpful, in the reassurance that couples gained from sharing with others who were going through a similar experience. The "sense of belonging" and the "strength to go on" were positive outcomes of group participation (Lentner & Glazer, 1991).

There are a number of groups that bear mention, as they can be helpful referrals for patients. Perhaps the best-known emotion-focused support group in the United States is RESOLVE, a national support group for infertility, which started in the kitchen of Barbara Eck Menning in 1973. The goals of RESOLVE at its inception were to help couples work through the anger and grief of infertility and to decrease their sense of isolation. Educating the public about infertility as a legitimate medical issue was also an early objective (Menning, 1976). Today, RESOLVE not only provides traditional emotion-based support groups but also hosts educational family-building conferences and has lobbied insurance companies to recognize infertility as a medical condition to cover treatment expenses. Other popular venues, known as *mind–body groups*, are based on cognitive–behavioral theory and incorporate a variety of psychoeducational components: relaxation training, nutrition and exercise awareness, cognitive restructuring, as well as emotional sharing and support (Domar, Seibel, & Benson, 1990; Domar, Zuttermeister, & Friedman, 1999).

There has been speculation as to whether psychosocial interventions actually increase pregnancy rates. In Boivin's (2003) review of the literature, it was found that although these interventions were indeed effective in reducing negative affect, pregnancy rates were unlikely to increase as a result of participation (Boivin, 2003). However, there is some evidence to suggest that mind–body groups not only decrease distress but also increase pregnancy rates (Domar et al., 2000). A study of infertile Japanese women, for example, found a higher pregnancy rate in those who had attended structured group interventions, which included psychoeducation, problem solving, relaxation training, guided imagery, and support (Hosaka, Matsubayashi, Sugiyama, Izumi, & Makino, 2002). Other research, however, has not found an increase in pregnancy rates (Chan, Ng, Chan, Ho, & Chan, 2006; McNaughton-Cassill et al., 2002). Clearly, more data are needed to fully understand the potential of psychological interventions on fertility. It is important for clinicians to realize that reproductive patients may do anything to increase their chances of pregnancy, and some may seek out these groups as a possible solution to their reproductive problems. Therapists need to help them clearly understand that although they may feel less stressed, less isolated and alone, and more prepared to cope, there is no guarantee that they will become pregnant because of psychosocial group interventions.

Although many people find support groups to be enormously helpful, they are by no means perfect or right for everyone. Some people are, by nature, very private and not comfortable sharing their personal lives with a group. Others become overwhelmed by the intensity of pain that can permeate these groups, as members process their experiences. If a person is at a particularly vulnerable time, he or she may find it difficult to be exposed to the stories of others in the group. Probably the hardest event that occurs in groups is when one of its members becomes pregnant (Covington, 2006). Although this is clearly the goal of all group participants, feelings of joy and jealousy are likely to collide. As happy as the group may be for the lucky couple, it may feel as if, once again, there is a division of sides: the haves and the have-nots. And although this is difficult for the members who are still struggling to reach their goal, it is also quite challenging for the pregnant woman as well. She may feel guilty about her success, not unlike survivor's guilt, and may worry that she is causing pain to the others. Within the group, tension or competitive feelings can also arise between members who have never conceived and those who have become pregnant but miscarry, as if, again, they are on different sides.

Whether the group is run by a peer or a professional, it is essential for the group leader to be acutely aware of these dynamics and prepared to address them. By giving voice to the various emotions, both positive and negative, that group members may feel when someone becomes pregnant, the leader opens the door to talk about these experiences; in so doing, she "makes the unspeakable, speakable," which traumatized reproductive patients so sorely need. The group becomes an in vivo example of what members deal with daily, when they are surrounded by friends, family, and strangers who become pregnant. The group venue, therefore, can be quite valuable; addressing these concerns in the safety of the group can help everyone learn to cope with similar issues in the real world (Covington, 2006). In addition, it is important for the leader to bring these issues up in a psychoeducational way early on in the group setting, advising members of what they might feel if someone gets pregnant, so that participants can be prepared (Covington, 2006).

It is also noteworthy, however, that some people build their lives around their support group, remaining involved or taking on leadership roles long after their own needs have been resolved. For some, this choice is generative in nature; it represents their way to give back to others the help that they themselves have received. These "veterans" can be invaluable role models for the other participants. In a pregnancy loss group, for example, seasoned members can provide hope for attendees. Because they are at a different stage in the grief process, newer members, who are fresh in their grief, can, in a sense, see into the future. They can understand that, over time, their grief will diminish; they will not always feel as devastated as they do now. The experienced members can demonstrate how their story and their grief have resolved—whether they have had a successful pregnancy, adopted, or remained a family of two.

On the other hand, a person who stays in the group during pregnancy or after may be fulfilling needs different from the most obvious ones associated with infertility or loss, and their presence may be uncomfortable for other group members. It is important that long-standing group members are aware of their own motivations for staying in the group. Are they having trouble making yet another identity shift, this time from infertility patient back to "normal"? Are they having difficulty grieving their prior loss and attaching to their current baby? Are they afraid to leave the group, having distanced themselves from their "pretrauma" friendships? Because these long-time members may not be in therapy, it can be helpful for the group leader to explain to new members some of the reasons that people choose to stay long after their trauma had resolved.

Jill, for example, was new to a support group for parents who had a pregnancy loss and became frightened when a long-time member shared the story of her loss. The loss, which had occurred 8 years earlier, seemed so fresh (the woman had been sobbing), that Jill wondered if that was how she would be in 8 years. She became frightened that she would never get over her own grief and was disinclined to return to the group. Jill discussed this experience with her individual therapist, who explained that the long-time member may have been in the group for reasons beyond grief over her loss and that her sobbing may have had to do with deeper personal issues triggered, but not caused by, the loss. Her therapist also took the opportunity to talk about the grieving process of continued bonds (as discussed in Chapter 5); she speculated that the group might provide the space, time, and place for this long-time participant to remember her baby. The therapist emphasized that the choice whether to continue the group or not was up to Jill. Although her patient chose to leave the group (realizing that she felt too vulnerable at this time to be exposed to these kinds of experiences), her therapist remained neutral about Jill's decision. The therapist knew, and reiterated to her, that if patients feel they are "supposed" to benefit from a support group and do not find it helpful, they may be left feeling, once again, that they are "not grieving right," adding another blow to their already fragile self-esteem.

INTERNET SUPPORT

It is hard to imagine life without the Internet. The amount of information that is literally at one's fingertips is staggering. These days, however, the Internet is not just a source of knowledge; it is also used to garner support for all kinds of medical maladies. Because infertility and reproductive loss are biopsychosocial experiences, the use of online support can fulfill patient's needs for technical and medical information, emotional guidance, and encouragement.

Online support is not unlike traditional support groups in content, focusing on emotional needs and providing information to its members. However, many prefer online support groups over face-to-face groups. In an exploratory study of online experiences, Malik and Coulson (2008a) investigated the perceived advantages and disadvantages of using an online support group, the affect it had on coping with infertility, and how it influenced the couple's relationship. They found that participants appreciated the ability to unload at any time of the day or night, liked the anonymity it provided (allowing individuals to ask questions or discuss issues without embarrassment), and felt a sense of control in that they could decide if and when to participate. Indeed, many clients, because of the sexual nature of procreation, or just because they are private people, are uncomfortable sharing their reproductive issues with family, friends, or in any face-to-face contact with a group. Because of feelings of shame or guilt, their natural support system may feel off limits. The safety and comfort of anonymous "sharing" allows individuals to gain support but maintain their privacy.

Malik and Coulson (2008a) found many benefits to the use of online support. First, it reduced the participant's sense of isolation. Many respondents felt that their family and friends did not fully appreciate what they were going through and found comfort in communicating with others who had firsthand knowledge of infertility. Because of the geographic locations of some couples, a "live" support group may not be available; in this case the Internet's function as a virtual-world network can be invaluable. Second, many participants also used their online group as a source of information. As mentioned earlier, they were able to ask questions without embarrassment and to use the information to empower them in discussing treatment options with their doctors. An interesting finding of this study is that participation in the support group may also have a positive effect on the couple's relationship. As one of the participants stated, "Having an online forum to visit helps me not to bombard my husband with conversations relating to infertility" (Malik & Coulson, 2008a, p. 108). Thus, having another arena in which to discuss feelings and garner support may decrease the strain and expectations of offline relationships.

Because women undergo the majority of the tests and procedures, even when the fertility issue is shown to be male factor, and because women tend to cope by reaching out to others for backing, it is not surprising that they are the largest users of online support. One study noted that 96% of messages posted were from women (Wingert, Harvey, Duncan, & Berry, 2005); another study reported that women made up over 98% of the participants (Himmel, Meyer, Kochen, & Michelmann, 2005). Women used the Internet primarily to gain information, ask advice, and elicit emotional support. The Internet has been helpful when used as a psychoeducational tool, reducing distress and increasing knowledge about medical decisions (Cousineau et al., 2008). Some women received continued emotional support by setting up and maintaining online relationships with others, establishing a "cycle buddies" group for help through a specific treatment cycle (Wingert et al., 2005).

Although it appears that women are the primary users of the Internet for infertility support, online forums have been shown to be helpful for men as well. Although women are more likely to share their feelings with their friends and partner equally, men often think of their partner as their only confidante (Jordan & Revenson, 1999). Because his partner is also struggling with the stresses of infertility, he may not want to impose his feelings on her, and he may feel it is his responsibility to be the stable force in the relationship (Dhillon, Cumming, & Cumming, 2000). Men are thus put in the position of suppressing their feelings. Online support groups can provide a safe, anonymous venue in which men can express emotions about infertility without embarrassment or inhibition. A study of men's posts on an infertility support group bulletin board revealed that men not only used the group to acquire information about medical interventions for themselves or their partner but also were able to vent their feelings openly, gain support, and obtain a much needed male perspective (Malik & Coulson, 2008b).

For those who have experienced a pregnancy loss, the Internet serves as a community of understanding parents with a shared grief. It is a virtual meeting place to discuss common themes: the attachment to their child during pregnancy, after the birth, and the continuation of this bond even after the child's death. Using others as support serves to normalize what otherwise feels so devastatingly lonely. Common topics that were found in online discussions include: the enormous sadness they all shared; the dread of holidays, birthdays, and due dates; the anxiety of subsequent pregnancy and fear of another loss; the use of meaningful rituals and symbols; and advice in dealing with siblings' grief (Capitulo, 2004).

As in face-to-face support groups, it is important to distinguish between monitored and unmonitored online groups. Many blogs and chat rooms are solely directed by peers, with no professional monitor or facilitator. In contrast, other online sites have specialists to answer questions in an "ask the expert" forum. The danger of unmonitored groups is that the information shared may not be accurate. Wingert et al. (2005) found that participants at times gave technical medical advice to other group members, without the guidance of a medical professional. Members of these groups who are looking for help may be at risk if they follow advice based on misinformation.

Patients who use monitored or expert forums often seek a second opinion online. Given the numerous options patients have regarding infertility treatment, it is not surprising that they would want the advice of another doctor; the convenience of doing this online is an added benefit of the Internet (Himmel et al., 2005). Interestingly, patients also used the monitored chats to bring up psychological problems. They expressed disappointment that they could not talk with their own doctors about their emotional state and complained that they were not treated as a whole person (Himmel et al., 2005). The implication of this finding is that, for most clients, there is a definite need for more psychological interventions during treatment. It is also logical that the Internet could be a potential venue to have some of these needs met. Although discussing the plusses and minuses of online psychotherapy is beyond the scope of this book, some of the obvious problems with online psychological counseling include the lack of confidentiality, boundary violations, and the loss of the ability to read body language, resulting in risk to the patient and increased liability for the therapist. As more is learned about the use of online counseling, it will be interesting to see if, in fact, it becomes a viable source of care for patients.

Although there are many positives to the use of online forums, there are negative aspects to these communities as well (Malik & Coulson, 2008a). As with live groups, hearing about (or in this case, reading about) other people's heart-wrenching stories can be overwhelming. The converse, reading about others' successes, can also be difficult for members. Whereas positive pregnancy tests can be a source of hope, they can also fuel despair in some individuals, so much so that people may withdraw from the group (Malik & Coulson, 2008a). Just as in face-to-face support groups, if it is addressed sensitively, a member's pregnancy can provide an opportunity for working through this painful and often times alienating period, for both pregnant and nonpregnant members (Covington, 2006).

Another downside is that some individuals may use the Internet to avoid real-world interactions, thus increasing their isolation (Epstein, Rosenberg, Grant, & Hemenway, 2002). It is not uncommon for people to become preoccupied and obsessed with their online community, thereby interfering with their daily life and relationships (Malik & Coulson, 2008a). From our clinical observations, the sheer amount of time patients spend searching for information and support can cause them to lose sight of time and perspective. Information can provide relief, but it can also increase anxiety and further questions or doubts. As we illustrate in the case of Patrice and Alex, it can create conflict in the couple's relationship as well, especially if one person avoids their partner by being online, or if they expect their mate to match their own enthusiasm for all they are learning. If the partner feels overwhelmed by the onslaught of information, he or she may withdraw, which the client can then misinterpret as abandonment or lack of caring. Last, caution should always be taken with the information and advice that is freely given out on the Internet, especially medical information, some of which may be inaccurate and potentially harmful (Malik & Coulson, 2008b).

As therapists have seen over and over, couples often cope differently with reproductive trauma, and the usefulness of Internet research and support will also vary within the couple. Some feel better if they can arm themselves with information, cover all their options, and stay connected with people in similar circumstances; others feel overloaded by this and prefer to follow their doctor's lead and not risk overexposing themselves to what they fear will be anxiety-provoking stimuli. If couples understand this, they can each benefit from the other's style: The one can share information with the other, and the other can help the one interpret the information and keep perspective.

As with any coping tool, however, the use of the Internet can become excessive and become a wedge between a couple. This happened to Patrice and Alex, a couple in their mid-30s, who dealt with their infertility—and the use of the Internet—in conflicting ways. Alex was very eager to have a child and felt quite optimistic that it would happen. He coped with any uncertainty by becoming more involved at work and other activities. Patrice, however, remained extremely anxious about her inability to conceive. She sought solace on the Internet, spending hours looking for information, trying to diagnose her medical problem, and comparing notes with others. Gathering information helped her feel less out of control and helped fill the time she spent waiting for each cycle to occur; she also found an online support group that was very helpful. Patrice also became very involved researching adoption; she was someone who needed a Plan B, even while preparing for Plan A. Alex, in turn, coped by staying busy and optimistic, focusing on their first IVF treatment, which was planned for the following month. Alex interpreted Patrice's time online as an obsession that seemed to him pessimistic and undermining; he worried that her incessant anxiety would compromise the IVF. It angered him to come home and find her ensconced on the computer. There were many nights when she did not come to bed with him because she was surfing the net; needless to say, this did not help their already fragile sexual relationship. He felt lonely and confused.

Patrice, too, felt frustrated; Alex seemed unwilling to talk with her about anything she was learning, and she felt burdened and alone, as if all the responsibility for mapping their path was on her shoulders. She sought reassurance online because she too worried that her anxiety would interfere with conception. Patrice aimed to discharge her anxiety constructively, by gaining information, guidance, and support. This was largely helpful to her, although she felt envious at times, when she spoke with women online whose husbands seemed more involved than Alex. The couple's therapist recognized a pattern in their relationship, common to many struggling with infertility: They were pushing each other away, each retreating angrily, in the face of what they perceived as rejection by the other. Patrice's use of the Internet increased, in part, because Alex was working more and seemed so unavailable to her, and Alex worked more, in part, because Patrice was always busy on the computer. The therapist pointed out to them that although each of their coping methods (work or Internet) could be helpful, when those methods became exaggerated in the face of hurt and anger, they became destructive rather than constructive. She encouraged each of them to set realistic limits on their time apart and to schedule specific times to talk about what each was feeling and learning. In this spirit, Patrice agreed to limit her time on the Internet and to postpone researching adoption until they found out the results of their impending cycle. For his part, Alex agreed to sit down with Patrice a few times during the week to review what she was learning and to discuss their options.

COMPLEMENTARY CARE

Alternative medicine has been in use for many conditions for a long time. Its popularity has grown in recent years, especially in the field of reproductive medicine. Individuals and couples often try many "natural" remedies to enhance fertility, including traditional Chinese medicine (which utilizes herbs and acupuncture), diet regimens and dietary supplements, yoga, and massage. Clients seek these adjuncts in the hope that it will enhance their chances of conceiving; the psychological benefit may come from the assurance that they have tried everything in their quest for a baby. And although some have had positive results (i.e., pregnancy), the research to date is not only limited but offers mixed conclusions. A brief review of the more common alternative medical treatment is discussed in the following sections.

Traditional Chinese Medicine

Perhaps the most frequently used alternative remedy is traditional Chinese medicine (TCM). Although it has been used to enhance human reproduction for centuries, there are limited controlled scientific studies that prove its effectiveness. It often relies on a combination of medicinal herbs and acupuncture to restore balance in the life energy or *Qi*, which flows through the body and universe. "It is the most indispensable energy that makes up the vitality of the body and maintains life activities" (Huang & Chen, 2008, p. 212). Qi has been defined as "inter-cellular information communicated within the body: information which enables all bodily functions and is a key component in regulation" (Ralt, 1999, p. 132). If this life force is blocked, disease will set in; to heal, the body must return to a healthy equilibrium. According to TCM, the kidney regulates not only the urinary system but the reproductive and endocrine systems as well; thus, kidney Qi must be abundant for a successful pregnancy (Huang & Chen, 2008).

With infertility patients, acupuncture is believed to increase blood flow to the uterus and ovaries, thus producing favorable uterine conditions (Westergaard et al., 2006). It has been recommended that acupuncture be administered once or twice a week for several months to improve reproductive deficiencies (Anderson & Rosenthal, 2007); however, it is often only used during IVF procedures before and after embryo transfer. Additionally, some Chinese herbs are used to activate blood flow (Huang & Chen, 2008).

With more and more patients wanting to utilize TCM for fertility treatment and to enhance IVF, many recent studies have been conducted to address its effectiveness. Some studies on women demonstrated that TCM increased pregnancy rates by increasing blood flow and energy in the uterus (Dieterle, Ying, Hatzmann, & Neuer, 2006; Paulus, Zhang, Strehler, El-Danasouri, & Sterzik, 2002; Westergaard et al., 2006). However, several other studies did not find statistical differences in the pregnancy rates between a group given acupuncture and a control group (Domar, Meshay, Kelliher, Wang, & Alper, 2006; Smith, Coyle, & Norman, 2006; Wang, Check, Liss, & Choe, 2005). There is also some question about the efficacy of using acupuncture before and after embryo transfer. In fact, one study found that pregnancy rates were lower for the group receiving acupuncture before and after embryo transfer than the control group, who underwent embryo transfer without any other intervention (Craig, Criniti, Hansen, Marshall, & Soules, 2007). Domar (2006) noted that in the Westergaard et al. (2006) study, the group receiving additional acupuncture after transfer had a higher rate of pregnancy loss than in the single-session acupuncture group, negating any positive effect of the treatment. Again, this kind of conflicting information may or may not be helpful to share directly with patients, who may not understand the intricacies and limits of any single research design. People tend to have a visceral reaction to such information that may not be applicable to their particular case. Whether or not acupuncture actually enhances fertility, many patients do find it very helpful as a way to relieve stress and anxiety. Making the choice to use acupuncture also allows women to regain a sense of control over their treatment and gives them a structured action that can help them tolerate the uncertainty of success and the agony of waiting for results month after month. In any case, therapists should encourage their female clients to check with their doctors before adding any supplementary herbs or acupuncture to their treatment regimen.

With male factor infertility, treatment with acupuncture two times a week for 5 weeks resulted in significantly improved semen quality, compared with a control group (Pei et al., 2005; Sherman, Eltes, Wolfson, Zabludovsky, & Bartoov, 1997). Another study, using a protocol of acupuncture twice weekly for 8 weeks, also saw a significant increase in sperm quality and fertilization rates (Zhang, Huang, Lu, Paulus, & Sterzik, 2002). A combination of acupuncture and Chinese herbal medicine also yielded positive results in treating men (Zheng, 1997). For enhanced sperm quality, it appears that acupuncture is a noninvasive, relatively benign treatment.

Because most of these studies have had relatively small sample sizes, however, there is concern that chance may play a part in the results (Collins, 2006). Reproductive patients are a captive audience and may be vulnerable to claims of success, even if concrete data are not available. Indeed, the placebo effect may play a role; the expectation that an alternative intervention will work may contribute to its success. Although this is not necessarily a negative consequence, it is important to tease out the effects of treatment from expectancy effects (Gutmann & Covington, 2006). More research is clearly needed to understand exactly how acupuncture and TCM produce physiological changes in both men and women.

Diet and Dietary Supplements

Research on weight and diet and their relationship to infertility has yielded interesting results, although more research is needed to thoroughly understand these interactions. When dealing with women at opposite ends of the weight spectrum, where the patient is either too thin or obese, the likelihood of irregular or absent menses is high. In very thin patients and those who exercise to an extreme, amenorrhea is a common occurrence. Anorexics may have low levels of luteinizing hormone and follicular stimulating hormone, which are related to anovulation and disturbance or absence of the menstrual cycle (Allison, Kalucy, Gilchrist, & Jones, 1988). It is thought that bulimia nervosa also results in hormonal dysfunction (Resch, Szendei, & Haasz, 2004). Similarly, ovulatory disorders are common among obese women. Indeed, one of the symptoms of polycystic ovary syndrome (PCOS) is excessive weight.

Depending on the condition (i.e., PCOS, anorexia), a change in diet may correct ovulation functioning, which in turn has a significant effect on a woman's ability to conceive. Often, severely underweight women can reverse their anovulatory state by increasing and maintaining weight above a critical level (Frisch, 1977). Likewise, overweight and obese women with PCOS benefited from either a dietary change or a structured exercise program (Palomba et al., 2008). A proposed "fertility diet," consisting of lower intake of trans fat and higher intake of monounsaturated fat, less animal protein and more vegetable protein, fewer glycemic carbohydrates and more high-fiber ones, more high-fat dairy products, and higher frequency of vitamin use, has been associated with a lower risk of ovulatory problems (Chavarro, Rich-Edwards, Rosner, & Willett, 2007, 2008). Over an 8-year period, Chavarro et al. (2007, 2008) examined women's dietary habits and found that the use of multivitamins, particularly folic acid, at least three times per week was associated with lower risk of ovulatory infertility. Because folic acid has also been shown to reduce neural tube defects (Czeizel & Dudas, 1992; Medical Research Council Vitamin Study Research Group, 1991), it has been recommended to pregnant women. Those planning to become pregnant may also benefit from multivitamin use (Chavarro et al., 2008). Patients should consult with their physicians before embarking on a particular diet or taking dietary supplements.

It is important that clients recognize that dietary changes do not guarantee success. As they might with any intervention, patients sometimes become obsessed with food, often depriving themselves to an extreme, in a perhaps misguided effort to enhance their fertility. Specific diets can be seductive to patients who feel compelled to try it as part of being thorough, even if it has nothing to do with their diagnosis. With so much of their life feeling out of control, strict adherence to a diet may be an expression of the client's effort to be in charge of what is happening to him or her. It can also turn into a type of self-punishment, which may speak to a patient's unconscious guilt or shame about their infertility or other aspects of their lives. As such, a client's decision to participate in extreme dietary or other lifestyle changes should be explored carefully in therapy, to ensure that it does not represent an unhealthy acting out of unexpressed thoughts or feelings.

YOGA, EXERCISE, AND MASSAGE

A belief held by many is that high stress and tension may cause infertility or pregnancy loss. There is no doubt that reproductive traumas create a great deal of anxiety for couples, but the question of whether stress is the *cause* is questionable. Relaxation techniques and exercise, such as yoga, are clearly beneficial to one's general health, but there is no evidence that they increase conception rates. One study examined the effects of exercise on IVF outcomes (Morris et al., 2006). They found that certain types of exercise patterns might affect live births after IVF. Specifically, women who reported exercising 4 hr or more per week for 1 to 9 years had less favorable outcomes than those who exercised between 1 and 3 hr per week for 1 to 9 years. Additionally, the type of exercise may make a difference, with cardiovascular exercise (i.e., jogging, running, aerobics, stair climbing, bicycling, elliptical training) having more of a detrimental effect than walking. The researchers speculated that shorter duration and less strenuous exercise may not be intense enough to alter hormonal functioning (Morris et al., 2006). It should be stressed that these findings are preliminary, and no clinical recommendations should be made on the basis of this one study; patients should always consult with their physician to determine what, if any, changes they should make in their exercise pattern. More research on the relationship between exercise, type of exercise, and conception clearly is needed to understand the physiological effects on IVF.

A massage technique based on physical therapy claims to open blocked fallopian tubes in infertile women. The intervention manipulates the peritoneum and uterine and ovarian ligaments to increase soft tissue mobility (Wurn et al., 2008). Others suggest that femoral massage, hip rotation, and deep tissue work may increase blood flow to the pelvic region, thereby increasing fertility. Although there have been claims as to its effectiveness, there are no studies to support these assertions (Gutmann & Covington, 2006).

SUMMARY

Reproductive patients are a vulnerable group. In their desperation to enhance fertility and increase their chances of a successful pregnancy, they are willing to try almost anything. Unfortunately, in the vast industry that reproductive medicine has become, patients may fall prey to unproven methods. It is critically important for both clinicians and patients to make the distinction between programs that claim to increase *pregnancy rates* and those that claim to increase *coping skills*. Because so much of patients' reproductive stories feels out of control, it makes sense for them to grab onto cures that may not have much evidence. Doing so gives patients a sense of empowerment. Although many of the alternative and adjunct medical protocols may be psychologically appealing, it does not mean that they necessarily increase conception rates or live births. Not only are more rigorous scientifically based studies necessary to know which treatments are most effective, but patients also need to guard against false assertions.

As long as a person's physician agrees that an alternative treatment is not detrimental and may provide an increased sense of coping, having patients pursue alternative methods is likely to be harmless. But patients should be aware that "one size does not fit all." Changing one's diet, for example, although prudent if one suffers from PCOS, is not a cure-all for all causes of infertility. The use of meditation, yoga, or acupuncture may also provide a feeling of control but may not alter the outcome of a cycle. Patients need to recognize that the specific problem they have may not respond to a particular therapy. The knowledge that they have tried everything can bring comfort, and as long as the particular intervention does not impair their chance of success, there is no harm in them trying it, with their doctor's approval. Many patients, after a failed cycle, will berate themselves for what they *haven't* done—as if that would explain the unsuccessful pregnancy attempt.

There is a popular notion that positive thinking will promote positive results. Clinical observation suggests that women often blame themselves for failed cycles because they were not relaxed enough or had negative thoughts. The self-blame that accompanies such thinking is destructive and promotes a downward spiral of negative affect. The mental health professional can address this self-recrimination by reminding patients that having a baby is a biological process and not one that is controlled by one's thoughts. Patients need to be reminded over and over that "conception is not a skill." Giving patients permission to express their anxious or negative thoughts actually provides relief—anything that is "unspeakable" gains in intensity, so verbalizing these thoughts makes them less frightening. If anything, suppressing or internalizing these negative thoughts causes physical stress and tension. It is especially important to remind patients that these negative or anxious thoughts are not only normal but inevitable, given the magnitude of their reproductive story and loss. Furthermore, although reproduction may be somewhat affected by stress, it is important to remember that women get pregnant during very stressful times—war, famine, or rape. If it were possible to control pregnancy by negative thinking, birth control would not be necessary! Reminding clients that they are not to blame is also a stress reliever, and, whereas this is not likely to increase conception, it will make them feel a lot better.

IV
ADDITIONAL CONCERNS

10

MEDICAL, MORAL, AND ETHICAL COMPLICATIONS

Given the fast pace of reproductive technology, choices that never existed before are open to couples. With these options come multiple psychosocial challenges and medical risks that can be difficult to navigate. Couples who embark on the use of assisted reproductive technology (ART) should be made aware of the potential problems, both medical and psychological, that they may face. For them to proceed with full informed consent, it is essential that the medical staff and/or mental health professional address the possible additional traumas that can occur during treatment. This chapter reviews these issues, with topics including:

- risk of multiple-fetal gestation,
- decisions regarding fetal reduction in a high-risk multiple pregnancy,
- death of a sibling in a multiple pregnancy,
- disposition of frozen embryos,
- use of technology to determine gender or other attributes, and
- secondary infertility.

MULTIPLE-GESTATION PREGNANCIES

Although women over 35 years old have a higher rate of conceiving multiples without fertility treatment, the number of multiple-gestation pregnancies has skyrocketed with ART and the use of ovulation-enhancing medication. By 1998, 56% of children born through ART were multiples (Centers for Disease Control & Prevention, 2002). From 1989 to 2002, the number of twin pregnancies increased 38.9%, which is more than 250% of the natural occurrence, while the number of triplets increased 172.7% (Evans, Kaufman, Urban, Britt, & Fletcher, 2004). These values are cause for alarm because of the far-reaching sequelae resulting from multiple births. There is a considerably higher risk of prematurity and low birth weight, as well as increased health risks to both mother and infants. Compared with singleton births, for example, cerebral palsy was found to be 4 times greater for twins; for triplets or higher, the risk was 17 times greater (American College of Obstetrics and Gynecology [ACOG], 2004). The cost, both emotionally and financially, of the treatment of children with major handicaps can be an onerous responsibility for the family as well as society. Additionally, the rate of infant mortality in the first year is much higher for multiples (ACOG, 2004).

For women, the medical risks associated with multiples can include gestational diabetes, hypertensive disorders, preeclampsia, placenta abruption, preterm labor, pulmonary problems, and caesarian births (Armour & Callister, 2005). These may in turn lead to other financial and emotional issues: loss of wages (because of required bed rest or hospitalization), increased feelings of depression, and the extra burden on the father to care for the woman and/or other children. Indeed, whereas the demands of taking care of one infant are enormous, when a twin (or more) is added, the need for help, as well as the expenses involved, rises exponentially.

With the medical and emotional price tag of infertility treatment as high as it is, many couples imagine that having a multiple pregnancy would be a perfect solution. In creating an "instant family," they would no longer be tied to the seemingly endless emotional and financial strains associated with ART. Although getting two (or more) for the price of one may seem like a good deal, the complications noted previously become much more significant with a multifetal pregnancy. Child, Henderson, and Tan (2004) asked men and women, independent of each other, who were undergoing infertility treatment to rate the desired number of children to have in one pregnancy. They found that 41% of all patients, regardless of gender, thought that having a multiple pregnancy would be ideal. Further analysis indicated that those who had been in treatment longer and still had no children were more likely to endorse the benefits of a multiple pregnancy. However, patients who understood the risks involved in multifetal pregnancies were less likely to endorse them as "ideal"

(Child et al., 2004). The importance of educating patients—by either the medical staff or mental health professionals—about the significant risks of carrying a multiple pregnancy is evident in these findings.

With the likelihood of having to endure multiple attempts at in vitro fertilization (IVF), many patients cannot readily afford treatment, and they, along with their doctors, must do a cost-to-risk analysis. The accepted belief has been that the odds of having at least one embryo "take" will be higher with the transfer of multiple embryos. Thoughts on this logic are changing, however, with more doctors opting to transfer only one embryo (known as *single-embryo transfer* [SET]), especially in women under 35 with good quality embryos, specifically because of the dangers involved. Interestingly, one clinic reported that, with the increase of SET, although pregnancy rates remained essentially the same, the incidence of twins dropped from 30% to 14% (De Sutter, Van der Elst, Coetsier, & Dhont, 2003). With ongoing technological advances and refinement, SET may prove to be even more effective in the prevention of multiple pregnancies in the future, especially with younger patients. For those over 35 years old, and for those who have been trying for a long time, the physical, emotional, and financial fatigue from numerous failed attempts may be enough reason to transfer more than one embryo. It is crucial, however, for patients to have a clear understanding of all the issues at hand.

The rate of multiple births in the United States is higher than anywhere else in the world. Speculation is that this is due to the lack of regulation of ART procedures in the United States compared with other countries. For example, Australia limits the number of transferred embryos to three, whereas in the United Kingdom, no more than two embryos may be transferred (Armour & Callister, 2005). While "success" is often measured by a positive pregnancy test, it does not take into account the potential difficulties that arise from multiple gestations: maternal medical risks, birth complications, neonatal care, and long-term consequences for birth-related conditions. The American Society for Reproductive Medicine (ASRM; 2009) has published guidelines on embryo transfer for clinics to follow, which take into account the patient's age, the quality of the embryo, whether there have been previous failed IVF cycles, and whether there are extra embryos to freeze. Although these recommendations are voluntary, allowing doctors to individualize treatment plans, it is suggested that patients under 35 with a good prognosis consider SET (ASRM, 2009).

Because of the risks involved, not just to the mother but to the child or children as well, it is essential that patients be truly informed about a multifetal pregnancy. The fact that patients are not mandated to see a mental health professional *prior* to using ovulation-enhancing medications or IVF means that they may already be pregnant with a multiple gestation when they seek the services of a therapist and have to make decisions about their pregnancy. Therapists can enhance clients' understanding of the risks involved in multifetal pregnancies and (as we discuss in the next section) can talk about the possibility of multifetal pregnancy reduction.

MULTIFETAL PREGNANCY REDUCTION

Multiple-gestation pregnancies present another dilemma for parents: *multifetal pregnancy reduction* (MFPR), also known as *selective reduction*. Because the threats to both mother and children increase with each multiple fetus, the choice must be made whether to maintain the pregnancy as is or opt for a reduction of the number of fetuses. Evidence suggests that reduction can lower the risk of complete pregnancy loss as well as severe prematurity (Antsaklis et al., 2004). MFPR also prolongs the length of the remaining pregnancy and thereby decreases overall health risks (Armour & Callister, 2005). Even in twin pregnancies, there is a better chance of taking home a baby if a reduction is performed (Evans et al., 2004). From a medical point of view, MFPR makes good sense, but it often presents agonizing moral and ethical quandaries for parents—and another loss, especially after struggling with infertility. Just as they are celebrating—finally—the achievement of a pregnancy, they must cope with yet another emotional choice: whether to reduce the number of fetuses (Collopy, 2004).

The decision to reduce a pregnancy can be extraordinarily difficult, especially if there is not a clear-cut medical need. Some decide ahead of time where they will draw the line: "I will carry triplets but not more . . . I will carry twins, but not triplets," and so on. But many people are not fully cognizant of all the risks associated with multiples and feel that "they can handle it, no matter what." Their thinking is that, having already gone through so much medical treatment to get pregnant, this circumstance is just one more thing they must get through.

People who have longed to have children for so many years may not be able to really process all the risks. "You hear it, but it doesn't mean anything, and the yearning for a child is so intense that it is hard to imagine that you might get more than you dreamed" (Collopy, 2004, p. 79). After so many losses, many couples assume that there is no way *they* would have to deal with a multiple pregnancy. Indeed, it is difficult for those who have been *in*fertile to imagine becoming *hyper*fertile (Collopy, 2004). Likewise, it is almost impossible for people to envision the reality of having premature births, so common with multiples, or the long-time sequelae that can burden such babies. Furthermore, as medical technology has advanced, the lower gestational age limit for surviv-ability has dropped considerably, increasing the number of babies who survive but also increasing the seriousness of the medical complications those children may present.

As with many aspects of work with reproductive patients, it can be exceptionally painful to sit with clients facing the decision about MFPR. Even when the therapist internally supports whatever decision is made, it is nonetheless a very difficult situation. It bears repeating that the therapist should remain impartial, supportive, and emotionally available during this process. The patients may be feeling enormously conflicted, and it is extremely helpful to have the sense that the therapist is there, steering the ship and keeping it from capsizing. The following case exemplifies the emotional upheaval that clients may face and the therapist's role in preparing them to cope with agonizing decisions.

CASE ILLUSTRATION: CARRIE AND SEAN

After 6 years of infertility treatment, including multiple IVF procedures and one miscarriage, Carrie and Sean were finally successful. At the first ultrasound, their doctor reported that the couple was going to have twins. In their therapy session following this appointment, although they were anxious about the risks of a twin pregnancy, they were also ecstatic and confident in their ability to cope. A few weeks later, however, they came to a session almost paralyzed by anxiety. At the second ultrasound, their doctor had detected another fetus. Suddenly, the couple was faced with the possibility of an even higher risk pregnancy, and the chance of all the babies surviving was now in question.

Sean and Carrie's feelings were all over the map. At one moment they felt confident that everything would be fine and she would be able to maintain the pregnancy. They worried that they might be "playing God" in making the decision to reduce. But they also acknowledged that it would be foolish not to recognize how dangerous it was to try to carry all three fetuses (Antsaklis et al., 2004; Armour & Callister, 2005) and that they might lose them all if they did not reduce. It was heartbreaking for them, but, after much discussion, Carrie and Sean opted to reduce the pregnancy from three to two fetuses.

Two days prior to the procedure, Carrie came to a session feeling overwhelmed and unable to think clearly. She described feeling frazzled, like she had to rush everywhere and had too much to do before the procedure. Noting her anxiety, the therapist asked her what was most pressing. "Well, I had this appointment today, and then tomorrow afternoon, I have my first well-baby check-up with the nurse practitioner, and then the next day I have to be at the hospital by 6 a.m."

The therapist was shocked. "How could Carrie put herself through a well-baby check now?" she wondered to herself, thinking how awful it would be to see the three babies the day before the reduction. "Is she feeling so guilty or angry that she has to punish herself?" The therapist asked Carrie if she had considered rescheduling the appointment with the nurse practitioner. "You are facing a very difficult experience. You have to detach from a baby that you worked so hard to create, in order to save the others. It seems torturous for you to go to that appointment, and endure seeing that fetus on the ultrasound with the others, knowing that you will terminate it the next morning. Why do that to yourself?"

Carrie looked stricken, and the therapist worried she had been too blunt. "I can't believe I never thought of that," said Carrie. "Thank you! I have been dreading tomorrow, but it never occurred to me that I could just reschedule it later. I feel so relieved. I have always worried that if I didn't do exactly what the doctors say, I wouldn't get pregnant, or they would be upset with me. I just thought I had to do what I was told even though it would be awful." Carrie had been feeling so guilty, with her emotions uncontrollable, that she was not able to rationally think about her plans. By canceling the appointment with the nurse, she was able to reclaim a small sense of control as well as protect herself from excruciating emotional pain. By labeling the guilt directly, the therapist also helped Carrie to see it more clearly; rather than the patient acting it out in a self-punishing way, they were able to talk about it. This allowed Carrie to see that guilt was a feeling, not a fact, and a feeling that she did not need to burden herself with. The therapist reiterated that Carrie had not sought out this situation; it was not her fault. She had never been thoughtless or careless. Indeed, the need to reduce was a trauma that was truly visited upon her, which she need not feel guilty about. This gave Carrie much relief, and she was able to follow through with the reduction in a much less agonized state. The doctor aborted the fetus that seemed the least developed; Carrie then carried twin sons to term.

After the birth, both Carrie and Sean were elated with their children, but they were nevertheless surprised at how sad they felt. When the therapist asked them to describe both sets of feelings, Carrie burst into tears. She explained that even though, intellectually, she knew they had made the right decision, she couldn't help but wonder about the baby they aborted. "I can't help but worry if that baby felt pain. And what if we aborted the wrong fetus? How can you choose? What if that was the baby that was meant to be born? What if she was my only chance for a daughter? I will never know what he or she would've been like." Carrie and Sean's reproductive experience started with infertility, multiple failed procedures, and a miscarriage. Conceiving triplets, followed by the unbearable decision to reduce, was trauma enough, yet they continued to be haunted by questions they would never be able to answer, no matter how hard they tried.

As Carrie and Sean demonstrate, making the choice to reduce is fraught with anxiety and trauma at many levels. Not only do couples have to process the experience themselves, but many are unsure about who they can trust or who they can turn to for help. How do they make this decision? Whom do they tell? What, if anything, do they tell the surviving children? Although the couple undoubtedly needs support, they may face unwanted criticism at a time they are feeling enormously vulnerable. Many clients avoid telling family and friends—the very people they would likely go to in times of need. Many fear reprisal or condemnation from their community for the decision to selectively reduce. For example, although Sean's family was more accepting, Carrie would never dream of telling her own family about the reduction. In fact, in all the years of treatment, Carrie had told no one about her infertility. As she worked through her grief at reducing the pregnancy, including her self-punishing plan to attend the check-up prior to the reduction, Carrie acknowledged how guilty and ashamed she had felt about her infertility all these years, which was then compounded by the need to reduce to twins.

Britt and Evans (2007a) distinguished four different styles of how people share their dilemma regarding reduction: *defended relationship*—only the couple knows what they are going through; *qualified family and friends*—sharing only with those who can be trusted; *both parents*—telling both sets of parents, regardless of their beliefs; and *extended network*—openly engaging others. They found that most couples engaged in more selective sharing (defended relationship or qualified family and friends) and that this gave the couples more of a sense of control. Whereas all the couples in this study understood the controversy involved in MFPR and felt considerable anxiety about it, those who were selective in their sharing felt more protected from the criticism of others (Britt & Evans, 2007a).

The procedure to reduce a fetus is done by injecting potassium chloride into the thorax of the fetus, thereby stopping cardiac activity (Antsaklis et al., 2004). Once multiple fetuses have been identified, at approximately 8 weeks gestational age, the couple has about 4 weeks to make their decision (Britt & Evans, 2007b). Although this may seem like a relatively short time, it can feel agonizingly long. During this time, the couple's worldview is truly tested. While under great stress, they must make an enormous decision that will have long-term effects on their family. And although discussing selective reduction prior to ART treatment may seem too early to some patients, sorting out their feelings beforehand allows couples to address the issue of MFPR in a less emotionally taxing way. Many couples complained that they had no idea the procedure even existed until faced with having to make a decision (Bryan, 2002).

Collopy (2004) found that women who were not told about MFPR in advance were shocked by getting the good news that they were pregnant with multiples at the same time that they were advised to reduce. Although the sample size in this study was small, the women who did not know about MFPR ahead of time declined to reduce. Conversely, those who were informed about MFPR earlier, during their infertility treatment, had time to digest the possibility, weigh the risks involved, and deal with their feelings, and were more likely to accept reduction (Collopy, 2004). This points to the necessity of patients being fully informed as they enter into ART, and it highlights the need for consultation with mental health professionals to help patients contend with the emotional and psychological issues brought up by reproductive technology.

Britt and Evans (2007b) analyzed the decision-making framework of women facing MFPR and found that patients used a combination of three underlying structures: *conceptual frame*—the belief that life begins at conception; *medical frame*—belief in the data and statistics demonstrating the benefit of selective reduction; and *lifestyle frame*—belief that women need a balance between children and career. As one can imagine, patients who had a strong conceptual framework struggled the most. Their belief that life begins with conception meant that ending that life, no matter how many other risks it posed, was morally wrong. Their focus was not necessarily on the fetuses that were to survive but rather on the sacrifice the other fetuses were making. In fact, some patients feel that MFPR is akin to murder (McKinney & Leary, 1999).

For patients with a high conceptual framework, the decision to reduce was most emotionally trying; other patients, however, had a comparatively easy time making this choice. Acceptance of the medical risks made the decision less difficult; thinking about the reduction as yet another one of the numerous medical procedures they had to endure to become parents took away the sense of guilt that others may have felt. Likewise, those who had another young child at home and knew they would not adequately be able to care for a multiple birth struggled less with the decision (Britt & Evans, 2007b). Carrie and Sean's initial response to the reduction fell into the conceptual framework; because of their long history of infertility, it was hard for them to consider ending a life they had created. They were able to resolve their guilt by acknowledging the medical risks involved in carrying triplets.

It is not surprising that couples struggle with MFPR. After going through so much to get pregnant, it seems like a cruel joke to have to then face termination of one or more fetuses. Couples may be torn within themselves as to what to do, but they also may have opposing views on this matter. Therapists can help guide the couple's decision-making process by understanding the ethical perspective of each member of the couple. Whatever decision the couple comes to, it is important that they are as comfortable as possible with it. Although the mental health practitioner will have his or her own belief system, which may conflict with the patient's, it is imperative to stay impartial. Here is another instance where countertransference feelings may run high (Bryan, 2002); the therapist's own reactions and decisions in this highly emotional arena may be counter to the decision of the patient. Keeping in mind what is best for the patient and child or children (American Psychological Association, 2002) can help quell the therapist's own anxieties about selective reduction.

LOSS OF A NEWBORN TWIN OR HIGHER LEVEL MULTIPLE

The mortality rate in a twin pregnancy (or higher level multiple) is much greater than with singletons (Scher et al., 2002). The rate of stillbirth in twin pregnancies is 3 times that of singletons (Bryan & Higgins, 2002); the higher the multiple the greater the chance of demise, either of the entire pregnancy or after preterm delivery (Bryan, 2002). As previously discussed, the rate of multiples, especially twin pregnancies, has significantly increased in the past decade because of the innovations of ART (Evans et al., 2004). Therefore, mental health professionals working with this population need to be prepared for the possibility of seeing patients who are coping with the demise of a twin or higher order pregnancy.

When none of the babies survive, the trauma to the parents is easily identifiable. The subsequent grief process is to be expected. When parents lose one baby but have one or more that survives, however, the emotional impact is confusing, overwhelming, and should not be underestimated (Withrow & Schwiebert, 2005). While they are grieving one infant, they must also attend to their live baby, who may be struggling in a neonatal intensive care unit. The contradiction of celebrating a birth and mourning the loss of a child at the same time creates enormous emotional confusion (Withrow & Schwiebert, 2005). Adding to the already complicated situation, these parents often receive little sympathy, even though they are grieving as intensely as if there were no surviving babies (Bryan, 2002; Swanson, Pearsall-Jones, & Hay, 2002). Friends, family, and even medical staff may suggest that parents should feel fortunate to have a surviving child. In their effort to assuage the parents' grief, they focus on the surviving child or children and try to persuade parents to do the same. This overlooks the need for the parents to grieve the baby (or babies) who has died, as well as focus on the one who has survived (Bryan, 1995; Wilson, Fenton, Stevens, & Soule, 1982).

Swanson et al. (2002) asked mothers what helped them at the time of their loss and what did not. Least helpful were insensitive comments such as, "But you still have one" or "You need to get on with your life" (Swanson et al., 2002, p. 161). Additionally, women complained that pressure from social workers to grieve in a certain way, lack of support from their partner, seeing other twins, medical staff who were not understanding, and blame—either self-blame or blame from others—were not helpful to them. Some of the factors that these women recommended for others who had lost a multiple included: not to isolate, join a bereavement group, avoid blaming themselves, create a bereavement ritual and name their babies, allow themselves to actively grieve, write about their loss, look for meaning in the loss—spiritual or otherwise, and seek medical and/or psychological help (Swanson et al., 2002). These are important suggestions for mental health professionals to keep in mind as they work with this population.

Sometimes the mourning of a multiple is delayed by months or even years because the parents are so preoccupied with caring for the surviving infant(s), especially if the survivor(s) is in critical condition (Bryan, 2002; Bryan & Hallett, 1997). If a parent does not grieve the loss, it may continue to fester inside of him or her. In some cases, parents may become overprotective of the surviving child or children, for fear of losing them as well (Bryan & Hallett, 1997), or they may fixate on or idealize the baby who has died (Withrow & Schwiebert, 2005). Mrs. J., for example, came for a consultation not because of a current reproductive issue but because she was worried about her 6-year-old son, Josh, who was withdrawn and had low self-esteem. As the therapist gathered Josh's developmental history, Mrs. J. revealed that Josh had been born 3 months early and had had a twin who died from medical complications in the neonatal intensive care unit. Mrs. J. believed that Josh's loneliness was because he somehow still missed his twin. As such, she had gone to great lengths to keep the lost baby in the forefront of their lives, "so Josh knows he has a brother." As she talked, Mrs. J. became flooded with sadness. It emerged that she herself continued to actively grieve the lost twin. This baby was frequently in the mother's conversation, which was a constant reminder to Josh—and to herself—that he had had a twin. When Josh came to therapy, it was not difficult to uncover his resentment at the constant comparison, his survival guilt that he had not died instead of his brother, and his low self-esteem as a child with a mother who idealized her lost baby and was unable to fully appreciate her surviving child. Enjoying Josh made Mrs. J. feel disloyal to her lost baby, yet holding on to the loss was exacting an emotional cost from Josh. In the parent work, Mrs. J. herself was able to recognize not only her guilt that she had been unable to save her baby but also her guilt over her wishes to focus on Josh and enjoy raising him.

Wendy presents another example of the emotional tug-of-war that parents feel. She became pregnant after her first IVF cycle with twin girls, and although she was aware of the risks involved, she was elated to have such good news after only one round of IVF. Aside from "enormous fatigue and gargantuan boobs," as she put it, the pregnancy itself was uneventful. At 35 weeks, however, she sensed something was wrong. One of the girls had had a cord accident, and Wendy delivered one healthy little girl and one who had died. Wendy was not sure what she was supposed to feel or do. Although she delighted in caring for Rose, she couldn't help but think of the lost twin, Lucy, at every moment. She was pulled in two directions at each turn: pleasure in caring for her surviving baby and shame that she was feeling this pleasure. She felt guilty for not spending the same amount of time and energy on Lucy; at these moments she could do nothing but cry. As she struggled with these conflicting feelings, it became clear that she needed permission to love both her babies but—and most important—that she had to love them in different ways.

These examples illustrate why it is so difficult, but important, to grieve the loss of a twin or other multiple. Validation of the unique process of this grief—the balance between celebrating and enjoying the survivor(s) while at the same time mourning the loss—is key in working with these families (Withrow & Schwiebert, 2005). Just because a parent is focused on the surviving child or children does not mean that he or she has abandoned the deceased child. In therapy, not only is it okay to talk about the baby who has died, but parents should be encouraged to do so because it is a necessary component of the mourning process. Parents may need to tell their birth story over and over again because this may be their only memory of their lost child. The difference between Mrs. J. and Wendy is that Mrs. J. had not allowed herself to fully grieve at the time of the loss; therefore, her conflicting emotions were unconsciously woven into her relationship with her surviving child, in ways that were not helpful to him. The therapist plays an important role as listener, especially if friends and family, who may be dealing with their own grief reaction, cannot tolerate the pain. Validating the discrepancy between feeling great joy and sorrow at the same time allows parents to work through these complex feelings.

DISPOSITION OF UNUSED EMBRYOS

A common side effect of IVF ovarian stimulation is the production of more embryos than can be used in one cycle. The remaining embryos are routinely frozen, often for the couple's future use in pregnancy attempts. However, couples who have completed their family and have remaining cryopreserved embryos must decide what to do with them. Currently, they may donate the embryos to another infertile couple, offer them for research, opt to have them thawed and destroyed, or destroy them by transfer to the mother when it is virtually impossible for her to conceive. This can be a highly emotional decision and is based on deep moral beliefs of how couples interpret the status of the embryo.

As of 2002, there were approximately 400,000 frozen embryos stored in the United States alone (Hoffman et al., 2003), with thousands more stored in Europe and Australia (Newton, Fisher, Feyles, Tekpetey, Hughes, & Isacsson, 2007). Although many of these embryos are targeted for the couple's own use, there are numerous reports of unclaimed embryos. If embryos are abandoned, IVF clinics are put in an uncomfortable position. Do they need to keep storing them, and if so, for how long? In 1996, the ASRM Ethics Committee (2004a) developed guidelines recommending that IVF programs procure instructions in writing from couples. This includes what to do with the embryos "in case of death, divorce, separation, failure to pay storage charges, inability to agree on disposition in the future, or lack of contact with the program" (ASRM Ethics Committee, 2004a). Their suggestion is that if more than 5 years have passed and after thorough attempts to contact the couple, it is reasonable for the IVF program to thaw and dispose of the embryos.

The fact that the Ethics Committee had to consider this issue is evidence of the struggle couples face in addressing surplus embryos. One woman spoke about her twins, now 16 years old, and their "siblings" that remain frozen because she is still at odds about what to do. Another couple originally had intentions of using their extra embryos after the birth of their twins but were surprised by a spontaneous pregnancy. Because they felt that three was enough, they too were left unsure of what to do about the remaining embryos. The irony of this situation is that at the beginning of IVF treatment, producing as many embryos as possible feels like a guarantee for success, but when child-bearing is completed, confronting feelings about frozen embryos can be emotionally and morally challenging. It is yet another affront to a couple's idealized reproductive story; the disposition of frozen embryos forces couples into ethical territory they never thought they would have to deal with when they first embarked on creating a family. Nachtigall, Becker, Friese, Butler, and MacDougall (2005) noted that many patients who had used an ovum donor had a more difficult time deciding what to do with their excess embryos than deciding to use a donor in the first place.

Although many clinics address the issue of surplus embryos at the start of IVF treatment, this is clearly not in the forefront of patient's concerns at that time. In fact, research has shown that patients change their mind about the disposition of embryos over time (Klock, Shenin, & Kazer, 2001; Newton et al., 2007). Studies have looked at this decision-making process: Results suggest that how parents conceptualized these embryos was key to their ultimate choice of donating to another couple, donating to scientific research, or having them destroyed. Some parents viewed their embryos as "virtual" children, whose welfare needed to be protected, whereas others thought of their embryos merely as biological material (De Lacey, 2007; Nachtigall et al., 2005). One would imagine that those in the virtual children group would have more difficulty destroying the embryos and be more inclined to donate them to another infertile couple; however, this was not always the case. They viewed their family as a biological unit, bonded together by genetics, and worried that the potential child would not be under their control. Donating embryos to another couple felt to them like relinquishing a child for adoption (De Lacey, 2007). They also recognized that, genetically, the embryos were siblings to their already existing children and were concerned about the possibility of consanguine relationships developing should another couple "adopt" them (Nachtigall et al., 2005). The parents who thought of their embryos as virtual children were therefore more likely to discard them (De Lacey, 2007).

In contrast, parents who conceptualized the embryos as biological material—cells or tissue—were more likely to donate them to another couple. Although it may seem counterintuitive—one would think that viewing embryos as inanimate cells would make it *easier* to destroy them—these parents opted to donate because they defined the relationships in a family as more important than genetics. In other words, they felt that the people who raised and nurtured the child were the *real* parents. Additionally, parents who donated believed that the *true* mother was the one who invested her body in the process of gestation and giving birth. Couples with this kind of emotional distance from their embryos, conceptualizing them more as a seed than as a child, were more likely to donate their embryos to another couple than have them destroyed (De Lacey, 2007).

The issue of stem cell research has prompted intense debate in recent years. Should stem cell research be limited to use of cells from adult lines only? Or is it acceptable to do research using surplus embryos? Once again, it is the interpretation of the status of the embryo that creates conflict over donation to scientific research. Some feel that embryos should be treated with the same ethical and legal rights afforded to living human beings; thus, destroying them for the sake of scientific advancement is not acceptable. Others assign them less evolved status. Donating them to stem cell or other research allows couples to feel that their embryos are not going to waste and that they are actually helping advance medical knowledge (McMahon et al., 2003; Zweifel, Christianson, Jaeger, Olive, & Lindheim, 2007).

Sue and Jess felt satisfied with the two children they had through IVF. When they first considered options for their spare embryos, prior to the births of their children, they seriously thought they would donate them to another couple. "We know, firsthand, how awful infertility is, and it seemed selfish not to want to help another couple." However, 4 years later, with seven embryos still remaining, Sue and Jess felt worlds apart from their previous ideas. They were uncomfortable with donating to another couple: Having their genetic material "somewhere out there" without their control and protection did not feel right. They were equally ill at ease just discarding them. "It seemed so wasteful. If we were not going to use them ourselves, and they could be put to good use, it seemed natural to donate them to a research program."

Sue and Jess's decision-making process is not unlike that of many other couples. It is common for couples to change their mind: How they think of disposition at the start of the IVF process often changes over time (Klock et al., 2001). At the start of treatment, patients are focused on getting pregnant and often have anxiety about producing any eggs at all. They are not in the mindset to think about disposing of something they are trying so hard to achieve (Lyerly et al., 2006). Understanding the dynamics of this process can help in the clinical setting. Nachtigall et al. (2005) suggested that couples go through stages in making this decision: (a) *reassurance* in large numbers of embryos at the beginning of treatment; (b) *avoidance* in thinking about the embryos once their family is complete; (c) *confrontation* with the need to make a decision; and (d) *resolution* if they were able to come to a decision.

Because thoughts about disposition change over time—several years usually pass from initial cryopreservation to eventual disposition—patients may need more counseling to reconcile past ideas with their current beliefs. Fully informed understanding of the process may not be possible until after medical treatment is completed (Newton et al., 2007). Although patients should have thorough knowledge about choices for embryo disposition before IVF, counseling should be offered on an ongoing basis until these decisions are finalized (Zweifel et al., 2007). In fact, Newton et al. (2007) recommended a two-stage consent process: one prior to treatment and again at the time of embryo disposition.

An additional complexity arises when the embryos in question are created using donor gametes. Ideally, the feelings and concerns of the donor should be addressed regarding embryo disposition, before creating the embryo. Legal contracts between recipient and donor need to speak to this sensitive issue. However, because many couples change their mind about what to do with excess embryos from the beginning of treatment to disposition (Klock et al., 2001), it is possible that a gamete donor, if consulted years later, might also change his or her mind about a specific disposition. Should the donor be sought out at the time of disposition? For example, should his or her permission be required if the recipients later decide to donate to stem cell research? Clinical experience with oocyte donors suggests that they are willing to donate to a specific couple but do not want their genetic material to be used by anyone else. Clearly, more research in this area would be helpful in providing guidelines that encompass donors' rights as well.

The disposition of cryopreserved embryos is complicated; couples forced to deal with these issues may feel the loss of their original reproductive story acutely, even if successful in their IVF attempts. Many feelings may emerge and change over time, and respect should be given not only to what patients want to have happen but also to what they don't want to occur (De Lacey, 2007). Some patients suggest having a ceremony at the time of disposal to honor the unused embryos (Lyerly et al., 2006). Whatever outcome clients choose, using the reproductive story as a metaphor can help them grieve yet another reproductive loss.

DESIGNER BABIES: SHOULD LIMITS BE SET ON EMBRYO TECHNOLOGY?

Preimplantation genetic diagnosis (PGD) is a technique that can be used in an IVF cycle to screen embryos before they are transferred into a woman's uterus. By removing one cell from the embryo, doctors can run tests to identify chromosomal abnormalities, and the results may be especially helpful for older IVF patients or patients with a history of miscarriage. PGD can also be used to detect susceptibility to disease, such as cancer or Alzheimer's. Additionally, parents who have a child who needs hematopoietic stem cell transplants may opt to use PGD for subsequent children, thereby ensuring that the next child is not only disease free but also can provide stem cells for the existing child (Robertson, 2002).

Aside from the medical uses of PGD, nonmedical uses—such as gender selection—raise considerable controversy. Is it ethical to choose an embryo on the basis of gender? Are there particular circumstances that make gender selection less problematic than others? If parents are "allowed" to pick their child's gender, might they eventually be able to select other traits, for example, height, hair color, athleticism, or intelligence? Should reproductive rights include these choices, or might this be harmful to society in general?

In many cultures, the "value" of a male child is much higher than that of a female child, especially the firstborn. In China, for example, male children are more desirable because they are perceived as more physically able and are expected to care for their parents in their old age. Because of China's one-child policy, the desire for a male offspring is high; consequently, many female children are relinquished for adoption. This has created an imbalance in the population, with Chinese men complaining of a lack of potential partners. As demonstrated by China's policy, the implication for society at large is an imbalance of the ratio of men to women (Hollingsworth, 2005).

One of the arguments against gender selection is that it deliberately produces embryos knowing that many will be destroyed. Once again, the status of the embryo comes into play: Should it have the same rights as a living child, or is an embryo inherently different? The attribution one makes will likely drive one's reproductive choices regarding gender selection. Although some may feel that gender selection is morally untenable under any conditions

(Watt, 2004), others contest that it is acceptable under certain circumstances. A specific gender may be preferred if a family already has a child or children of the opposite sex. "Gender balancing," as it is commonly called, was initially discouraged by the ASRM Ethics Committee (1999), but later the committee suggested that it would be acceptable as long as it was not for the first child (ASRM Ethics Committee, 2001). In cultures, such as India, in which a male heir is of utmost importance, using PGD in a family that already has a daughter may be considered morally acceptable (Robertson, 2003).

When one thinks about the premise of the reproductive story, and all the hopes and dreams that parents have for their offspring, it is reasonable to expect that parents want the best for their children. Many parents take great steps and make financial sacrifices to provide for their child's education and welfare. If a person wants his or her child to thrive, it makes sense that he or she would want to pass on the best of his or her genes. With knowledge derived from the Human Genome Project, it may be possible in the future to identify certain personality traits that could allow parents to reject embryos based on nonmedical concerns. The fear is that this will lead to a society based on eugenics, putting those who have the financial means to use PGD, or other like techniques, at an advantage. Although the technology is not available right now, it is not far-fetched to think of a time when selection of specific characteristics in an embryo would be possible (Galton, 2005; Hollingsworth, 2005). How this will play out in the future, and what legal interventions governments will employ, remains to be seen.

SECONDARY INFERTILITY

Primary infertility is generally defined as the inability to conceive or carry a pregnancy to term after 12 months of unprotected sex. *Secondary infertility* is the inability to achieve a pregnancy after already having one or more children. In the United States, the proportion of women with secondary infertility (70%) is higher than primary (30%), perhaps because women seeking a second child may be older than those trying to conceive for the first time. Women with primary infertility, however, are twice as likely to seek treatment, compared with women with secondary infertility (Hirsch & Mosher, 1987). The research on the psychological adjustment of this group is sparse, in spite of the disproportionate number of women with secondary infertility. Although this group has high levels of emotional distress (La Joie, 2003), most studies focus on primary infertility.

Those suffering from secondary infertility are in a unique position and may feel more isolated because of it. Where do they fit in? They are technically not part of the infertile world—after all, they have succeeded in having at least one child—but they are also not part of the fertile world because they struggle to have another baby. They may be misunderstood by support groups dealing with infertility and may feel out of place with other parents, especially those who are pregnant with another child. They may be getting the message from the infertile world that "one should be enough," whereas the fertile world suggests that "two (or more) is better."

Anecdotal evidence suggests that women with secondary infertility feel enormous guilt and shame about their special circumstances. One woman, at an infertility conference, felt intimidated about asking a question and only approached the speaker after the session was over. Rightfully or not, she didn't feel she would get the understanding of the group, who were all struggling to have their first child. Although primary infertility patients feel as if they are on one side of the fence with the fertile world on the other, secondary infertility patients feel as if they are straddling the fence and have no solid ground to land on.

Women with secondary infertility may also question their own identity and status: Having already had a child, they may not believe they have infertility and therefore don't seek treatment. Defining oneself as having fertility issues may be so distasteful that denial of the problem—even though medical and psychological treatment may help—feels emotionally safer. Women with secondary infertility may also be less likely to seek services if they had previously been diagnosed with primary infertility. Having already experienced the trauma of treatment, they may be less inclined to walk down that road again. More research examining the unique emotional features of women and couples with secondary infertility is necessary.

As they raise the child they have, patients with secondary infertility may also be caught off guard by recurrent grief feelings that may come up at unexpected times. Tara, the mother of a 4-year-old son, had truly felt that she had come to terms with her secondary infertility. She was having a wonderful time raising her son and looked forward to the future as he grew. When he started preschool, however, a milestone that she had anticipated with pride and excitement (and a touch of nostalgia), she became inexplicably depressed. She became reluctant to drop off or pick up her son, asking that her husband take over that task. In analyzing this avoidance, Tara realized why it was so painful for her to be at the school: So many of the other mothers were either pregnant or had infants in addition to their preschooler. Seeing these families had reevoked images of her reproductive story, fantasies about the sibling she had planned for her son, and sadness about how her story had changed. By allowing herself to grieve anew, at this stage of her son's life, Tara could set the feelings of loss in the background and resume her enjoyment of her family's life. This is an important reminder to therapists that the grief process is not linear or time limited and does not always occur during the immediacy of the reproductive trauma. Tara showed that grief waxes and wanes as circumstances dictate, and patients need to be reassured that the resurgence of grief at unexpected times is normal.

SUMMARY

The medical advances in ART over the past several decades have outpaced the understanding of the psychological, ethical, and moral ramifications of its use. Although couples are eager to try these new medical options, they can be overwhelmed by the many unanticipated consequences. Knowing the "side effects" of ART is an important part of helping patients cope with their emotional reactions. As the technology continues to grow, more questions will likely arise; it is the mental health practitioner's role to stay up to date with the continually changing landscape and the natural emotional corollaries that follow.

11

PREGNANCY AND PARENTHOOD AFTER INFERTILITY OR REPRODUCTIVE LOSS

It would be wonderful to start this chapter by saying that the trauma of infertility and reproductive loss simply disappears once a baby is born. Although much healing can and does take place following a successful pregnancy or adoption outcome, research has noted that a history of reproductive loss or infertility is associated with increased anxiety during pregnancy, often related to fear of another loss and pregnancy demise (Brockington, Macdonald, & Wainscott, 2006). Although there are many overlapping feelings about pregnancy postinfertility and postperinatal loss, these are addressed separately; the focus of patients' attention, as will become apparent, is often different. Additionally, this chapter addresses postpartum reactions, which can occur even when a baby has been very much desired and hard sought after. This can be difficult for people to understand; they may feel added shame that, after so much effort, they are still not happy, and they may be resistant to seeking treatment. As such, it is important for mental health practitioners in this field to be able to diagnose and treat postpartum adjustment difficulties.

PREGNANCY AFTER INFERTILITY OR REPRODUCTIVE LOSS

Pregnancy Postinfertility

When clients at long last achieve their goal of becoming pregnant, the assumption is that all the pain and suffering from the trauma of infertility will vanish and happiness will abound. It can be quite startling to patients, and to their friends and family, when their moods continue to be fraught with anxiety and depression. The initial jubilation they experience may be replaced with worry and apprehension. The transition from infertility to pregnancy can be frightening for these patients: The fear of losing the pregnancy is paramount. These clients have already suffered from so many losses that they are convinced another loss is inevitable. If they have used assisted reproductive technology to conceive and have seen the embryos developing, or viewed their first ultrasound, they may be thrilled at observing their family-to-be, yet at the same time feel a need to distance themselves from the reality of pregnancy. They may be wary of getting too attached—"cautiously optimistic" is heard time and again in the clinical setting—and some may even deny they are pregnant, continuing to identify themselves as infertile, afraid to believe their ordeal is over (Sandelowski & Pollock, 1986). This is not unlike the combat veteran who continually worries that danger is still just around the bend. Steeling themselves against loss may create its own sense of loss—the loss of feeling pleasure at finally achieving a pregnancy. One woman described this poignantly: "I have looked forward to this for so long. I should be happy; I *want* to be happy. But instead, I am constantly worrying. Every time I go to the bathroom, I do this mental dance, preparing to see blood from a miscarriage. It's like I can't bear to risk being taken by surprise if I *do* miscarry, so I am constantly on guard for it. It makes me sad, that even now, when I am finally pregnant, I can't enjoy it the way my friends enjoy theirs."

Another phenomenon that occurs with the postinfertile patient is that they must process yet another shift in their identity. As discussed previously, infertile patients experience an initial shift in their sense of self from "healthy, normal, fertile" to "infertile." That shift, at the beginning of treatment, requires a major adjustment in self-concept: They often feel betrayed by their body ("it's just not working right") and become so consumed with treatment that they ignore the other valuable parts of themselves. It is quite common to feel left out of the fertile, child-centered world; instead, new relationships develop based on the camaraderie shared with others going through fertility treatment. But suddenly they feel thrust out of that world as well. They must redefine themselves again, but how? They are still not yet parents (and remain fearful that they never will be), but they have definitely crossed over the "fertile line." They may be afraid of hurting their infertile friends, may feel guilty of their new status, yet they are not quite ready to invest in their own pregnancy that might yet be lost (Sandelowski, Harris, & Black, 1992). As one patient stated, "I have spent so long trying to *get* pregnant, that I don't know quite how to *be* pregnant. I don't know who I am anymore." This is a refrain we hear over and over again from patients going through treatment.

Infertility patients also lose the attention of the reproductive endocrinologist and staff once they "graduate" from their care. Patients may have seen their doctor or associates almost daily for months or even years, but when they continue pregnancy treatment with their regular ob–gyn, they go from being treated as a "special case" to a "normal pregnancy" (Sandelowski et al., 1992). This change can be most disconcerting: How can they be considered normal after all they have been through? The new doctor may not realize how intensely anxious they are—that they feel far from normal—and why. Furthermore, not only do they miss the attentiveness of the infertility specialist but many people also become very attached to their doctors and miss them greatly when it is finally time to say goodbye. Although it can be helpful to remind clients that they can go back and visit their doctors, that may or may not be comforting: Once they finally leave, they may find that returning to that office ends up retraumatizing them, reminding them of all they went through. It is important for therapists to normalize the ambivalence that clients feel during this transition, so that they will not view it as yet another thing they are doing wrong.

In this limbo state, the formerly infertile patient may feel at odds with both the fertile and infertile world, adding to a sense of isolation. Rather than identifying with either, they feel as if they are straddling both (Olshansky, 1990). Sometimes, this is intensified by their sensitivity to other infertile couples, in not wanting to foist their pregnancy on them. "It was so hard to tell our support group that we had a successful cycle, even though that's what we all hope for, for everyone in the group," said Sara. "I was reluctant to tell them, because I knew how painful it would be." Sara's feelings typify what many postinfertile clients struggle with: They want to embrace the pregnancy and share their good news with others, but at the same time they fear becoming attached to the pregnancy, are concerned they may hurt their infertile friends, and worry that those who are still struggling with infertility will reject them. The postinfertile need to relinquish or "let go of the negative identity, feelings, and thought patterns developed in the course of the struggle to conceive" (Sandelowski et al., 1992, p. 288), but this is not an easy process. In a sense, postinfertile couples need to grieve their infertile status in order to accept their pregnant state, just as they have had to grieve each of the previous shifts in their identity; they once again lose a sense of belonging and the paradoxical comfort of what has become a familiar, if not desired, state of being. When Sara finally told the group, she was relieved by their warmth and acceptance; they did not want to lose her friendship either.

The method of conception may also influence the adjustment to pregnancy. If a couple conceives using donor technology, for example, they must grieve the shared biological connection with the child. Other medical interventions, such as in vitro fertilization (IVF), increase the odds of having a multiple pregnancy, as well as the risk of prematurity, bed rest, and other medical complications (see Chapter 10). The shift in identity—from infertility patient to pregnancy—is thus done in a stressful, risky, and costly context (Sandelowski et al., 1992).

Pregnancy After a Perinatal Loss

When a baby dies in utero or shortly after birth, the loss is like no other. Death out of the natural order (i.e., parents predeceasing grandparents, children predeceasing parents), death when there was no chance to know and nurture the baby, death when there should have been life—there are no words to describe the devastation. Women often feel responsible, wondering what they did to deserve this, as if their actions or inactions caused the demise. Some conclude that their uterus was not the safe haven it was supposed to be, fueling the blow to self-esteem and the sense of inadequacy that so many reproductive patients experience. Other women describe the feeling that there is a hole inside them, never to be filled again, or that their arms literally ache with the longing to hold their baby. The physical sensation of emptiness is accompanied by the emotional state of futility and hopelessness. Men also feel a sense of emptiness: As Richard described it, "I keep thinking that my wife is still pregnant. Where is my little girl? I was so ready to spoil her and treat her like a princess . . . but now she's gone. I don't ever think I'll be the same again." Truth be told, he never will be the same again. Although Richard's grief will evolve and subside over time, as discussed in Chapter 5, it can take a very long time to come to grips with a pregnancy demise. The loss of a baby does change people, and it will impact the rest of their life.

Some feel that the only way to heal from this devastating loss is to have another child as soon as possible. The idea that the birth of another infant will negate the pain of the loss is a common, but misguided, notion. Indeed, the advice that is freely handed out is "You're young, you can have another" or "When you have another baby, you'll feel better." The implication is that one baby can replace another without issue. Not only does this minimize couples' grief, but it also suggests that the attachment to the lost baby is meaningless. A subsequent pregnancy does not erase the loss.

Although the term *replacement child* has been used in the literature to describe the conscious decision to have another child subsequent to a perinatal loss (Cain & Cain, 1964), this phrase adds to the assumption that one baby can simply be "swapped" for another. The experience of parents' grief, however, establishes that this is not so. Reid (2007) noted the complexity of emotions following a loss and subsequent pregnancy. Mothers do not want to replace the child who was lost; they simply want that child back. Rather than feeling they are replacing the infant with another, they hold the real or imagined view of the deceased as a template for the subsequent child. The term *penumbra baby* (or *shadow baby*) is perhaps more adequate to describe a subsequent pregnancy: The next child is "born in the shadow of the lost infant rather than as a replacement" (Reid, 2007, p. 182). This can have serious consequences for the subsequent child, in having to live up to the image or ideal of the dead child.

Pregnancy after a perinatal loss is likely to be filled with anxiety and posttraumatic stress disorder (PTSD)-like symptoms (Born, Soares, Phillips, Jung, & Steiner, 2006). Patients wait for what they feel is inevitable: a repeat of their previous loss. Waiting for "the other shoe to drop" heightens awareness and comparisons between the two pregnancies. They are hypervigilant to signs of another demise, especially around the time in the pregnancy that their previous loss took place. Clients may try to "do" the subsequent pregnancy differently. If the baby who perished had been a boy, for example, they may hope for a girl, so as not to repeat their loss. One woman refused to shop in a particular store during her subsequent pregnancy, as she had first experienced cramping there during the previous pregnancy.

It is normal for women to have a difficult time bonding to the new pregnancy (Reid, 2007). They feel detached and guarded as a self-protective mechanism. In their attempt to ward off the pain of another demise, they express guilt over not connecting with their current fetus, but they may also feel guilty feeling that they are abandoning their previous baby for the new one. In working with these patients, it can be helpful to give them "permission" to love both. They do not have to reject one infant in order to be loyal to the other. Letting patients know that it is possible both to grieve the past and embrace the future at the same time can help them through this anxious period.

Although most of the research has focused on women's reactions, it is critical to also recognize the psychological impact on men of pregnancy following a perinatal loss. Fathers as well as mothers experience considerable levels of anxiety during a subsequent pregnancy (O'Leary & Thorwick, 2006; Turton et al., 2006). Men may feel a need to be strong and supportive of their partner; thus, they tend to hide their own anxiety. O'Leary and Thorwick (2006) found that the "overt behavior [of men] contradicted their inner state of stress and vulnerability" (p. 81). Their needs are put aside to protect their partner, as evidenced by an increased watchfulness over the health of the mother and baby (Armstrong, 2001). With the subsequent pregnancy, men coped by checking in on their wives more often, making sure that she could still feel fetal movement. Societal expectations played into the role men assumed as well. Others, including health care providers, take for granted the supportive role men play; consequently, men's underlying emotions often go unrecognized, regarding both the grief of the previous pregnancy loss as well as the anxiety during the subsequent one (O'Leary & Thorwick, 2006). Because the outward expression of men's grief is often not socially accepted, it may emerge as increased use of alcohol or prescribed medication (Turton et al., 2006), preoccupation with work or other tasks, or anger and avoidance (O'Leary & Thorwick, 2006). It is especially important for the mental health clinician to look for these symptoms in men, acknowledge their difficult position in needing to be the support system for their partner, and provide an outlet for the release of their negative emotions.

PARENTHOOD AFTER INFERTILITY OR REPRODUCTIVE LOSS

Parenthood Postinfertility

What happens when a baby is born after infertility? Does the negative impact of infertility trauma simply disappear? Or are there longer lasting effects that continue on into parenthood? Although it is well established that infertile patients have higher levels of anxiety and depression, which often continue through the pregnancy, does this translate into negative reactions postpartum? What if the infertile couple adopts? Does adoption also mitigate the effects of infertility?

It may be assumed, after "surviving" infertility and having a child, that parents' emotional response would be happiness and a sense of relief. Although they may be overjoyed with at long last achieving their goal, there is a range of emotions that affect the formerly infertile, whether they achieve parenthood through childbirth or adoption. Certainly elation is one response, but just as all new parents must make the adjustment to sleepless nights and the demands of a newborn, so do those who had been infertile. One of the differences, however, is that the previously infertile feel guilty admitting to any less than enthusiastic feelings about their newborn. Having worked so hard at having a baby, these new parents don't feel they have the right to complain. The social expectations that they *should* be happy may cause women to censor any negative emotions (Olshansky, 1995). The idealization of themselves as perfect parents with a perfect child makes any expression of negativity seem ungrateful (Garner, 1985).

Abbey, Andrews, and Halman (1994) investigated the effect of parenthood postinfertility. Their study found that parenthood increased the global sense of well-being in infertile women who had become pregnant, compared with infertile women who did not become pregnant. However, in terms of their marital satisfaction, parenthood had a negative effect on formerly infertile couples, with less intimacy and sexual frequency. Interestingly, women who had no problems conceiving also experienced less sexual intimacy and frequency after they had a child but did not experience greater global life quality. It would seem, from these results, that parenthood does mitigate many of the negative effects of infertility while causing other effects that are common to *all* new parents: fatigue, less leisure time, and less time and intimacy with one's partner. As these researchers noted, it is helpful for health care providers to prepare their formerly infertile patients for the normal stressors of parenting an infant (Abbey et al., 1994). Letting them know that it is perfectly acceptable to feel ambivalent or complain about their newborn can reduce their self-criticism and can actually allow them to enjoy their baby more.

Infertile couples who become parents through adoption face other challenges as well. By the time a couple decides to adopt, they are already exhausted by the trials of infertility but must be ready for yet another difficult process. Adoption is often seen as the last resort for patients and, because of this, they must, first and foremost, grieve the loss of a biological connection to their child or children. The narcissistic wound of infertility should be healed and mended as much as possible prior to adoption. The goal for parents who adopt is to actively *choose* adoption rather than passively *resign* themselves to it.

Although research indicates that adoption does reduce the pain of infertility (Daniluk & Hurtig-Mitchell, 2003) and that adoptive parents and their children often have better adjustment than biological parents (Borders, Black, & Pasley, 1998; Levy-Shiff, Bar, & Har-Even, 1990), it is not a simple decision. An identity shift—from biological to adoptive parent—must occur for parents to embrace this decision (Daly, 1989; Sandelowski, Harris, & Holditch-Davis, 1993). Often, one partner is more ready than the other to forge ahead, and this can create tension in the relationship. Not only must clients come to grips with their own sense of loss, they must also negotiate with their partner so that both enter the adoption process in agreement.

Most adoptive parents must undergo an assessment of their home, character, and marriage to assure they are "suitable." Many feel insecure and anxious that they will not be chosen by a birth parent. The vulnerability they feel in putting their future parental status in the hands of a birth parent or an agency can feel humiliating and judgmental: They feel they are "on display" and "need to sell themselves." The uncertainty of if and when they might be selected—selection often takes years—adds to their sense of helplessness and anxiety. This anxiety often persists with the worry that the birth mother will change her mind and want her baby back. Parenting an adopted child also must take into account the ongoing relationship with the birth parent or parents and often the birth grandparent(s). The amount of "openness" in the triad of the child, the birth family, and the adoptive family varies, but how this is managed is yet another challenge that adoptive parents face in raising their child or children. In the case of international adoptions, where there is often very little information about the biological parents, adoptive parents have the additional task of helping their child understand their unique origins and incorporating the child's heritage and culture into the fabric of his or her life.

Perhaps one of the most difficult decisions for preadoptive parents to address is their willingness to accept a child when there are questions about the lifestyle of the birth mother or the health of the baby. After trying so hard to have a child, they may make negative assumptions about any birth mother who would relinquish a baby. Adoptive parents also worry about the prenatal environment: They are not in charge of the pregnancy (as they would be if they themselves were able to conceive), and they cannot control the birth mother's diet or her use of caffeine, cigarettes, drugs, or alcohol. Is a child born with genetic anomalies or addictions someone the adoptive parents can accept and are equipped to deal with? Additionally, adoptive parents need to confront their biases and consider their feelings about raising a child who is of a different race and/or culture, if one is offered to them. Not only must they think about their own feelings, but they also need to bear in mind what it means to the child to be a part of a mixed-race family. Adoptive parents must go beyond the normal duties of parenthood—such as nurturing, caring for, and educating their children—and understand the unique physical and/or psychological needs of their adopted child (Santona & Zavattini, 2005).

Even after successful resolution of infertility, by biological or adoptive means, it is important to note that parents may still feel the effects of infertility. Couples may have *delayed grief*, defined as a grief reaction that may occur weeks or even years after the initial loss or trauma (Middleton, Raphael, Martinek, & Misso, 1993). These feelings can be confusing: Why should they be unhappy now, when they finally have a baby? But clinical observation reveals that sometimes it is only after a child, whether biological or otherwise, is in their arms that individuals can allow all the feelings of their past trauma to emerge. They have been in "survivor" or "warrior" mode for so long—coping with surgery after surgery, procedure after procedure, loss after loss—that they haven't been able to recognize or acknowledge how far off track their reproductive story has gone; it is only after the crisis has passed that they can look back at the roller-coaster ride they had been on.

The following sections define adverse postpartum reactions and describe why they can occur after a reproductive trauma, for new mothers as well as fathers, whether they gave birth or adopted their baby.

POSTPARTUM ADJUSTMENT

Most parents-to-be have an idealized view of their baby and what parenthood will be like. The typical reproductive story includes images of contentment, happiness, and love for a new and adorable baby. Postpartum depression (PPD), however, is a widespread disorder that often goes undiagnosed and can include severe anxiety attacks, obsessive thinking, guilt, suicidal thoughts, or doing harm to the baby. It is estimated that it affects one in seven new mothers (Wisner, Chambers, & Sit, 2006). The experience can be shocking to new parents—nowhere in their reproductive stories did they expect this—and because of this, they often deny or misinterpret their symptoms and do not seek help.

Many disorders may get lumped into the category of PPD, but each should be differentiated for proper diagnosis and treatment. *Postpartum blues* or *baby blues* is a relatively mild reaction occurring within the first few days after birth. It may include tearfulness, fatigue, anxiety, and irritability and usually resolves after 10 days postpartum (Beck, 2006). Although the symptoms are not acute, it is estimated that 60% to 80% of women experience postpartum blues (Vieira, 2002). Because of its lack of severity, many health care providers, as well as the women themselves, dismiss the blues as a normal part of childbirth (Olshansky & Sereika, 2005). Indeed, it may be a reaction to the enormous hormonal shift a woman experiences after giving birth. Postpartum reactions, however, are more than biologically driven; theoretical models reflect the biopsychosocial aspects of the postpartum period (Boyd-Bragadeste, 1998). It is not just hormonal changes that affect a woman but also changes in her lifestyle (i.e., having to care for an infant), in her identity (i.e., taking on a new role as mother), in her social environment (i.e., going from a working woman to a stay-at-home mom), and/or changes in her relationship (i.e., shift in expectations and time spent with her partner).

Because women often hide their negative feelings postpartum, due either to shame or fear that they will be judged, health care providers may miss the postpartum symptoms. Although this may not be significant for women whose blues resolve, it is alarming that those with more serious depressive or anxious symptoms also minimize them. They may feel guilty for having and expressing these feelings (Gruen, 1993), but the risk of not doing so and not seeking professional help can endanger their child, their relationships, and themselves.

Postpartum anxiety can present as panic attacks in new mothers who had never had them before; as obsessive–compulsive disorder with ruminative thoughts of harming the baby or intense and unrealistic worry about the baby; or as PTSD, often after a particularly difficult birth. Some research suggests that postpartum anxiety is actually more prevalent than PPD (Brockington et al., 2006). Although plagued by obsessive thoughts, women with postpartum anxiety are confident that they will not act on their negative thinking. Unlike postpartum psychosis, these women recognize that their thoughts are irrational and know that hurting their baby would be wrong (Beck, 2006). Their anxiety and compulsive behaviors may, in fact, be related to worries that something will harm their baby and that they are not competent to protect their child. One woman, for example, slept under her baby's crib, fearing something terrible would happen during the night. Another woman insisted that the baby, who was quite healthy, have a monitor on in case the baby stopped breathing. Some women's anxiety may be serving them as a defense against negative feelings toward their newborn. These women may project their ambivalence onto their infant and then protect the baby from their own hostile fantasies by excessive worry. For these patients to receive the appropriate treatment, it is important for the mental health practitioner to discern the true source of their anxiety.

Of the women who experience the blues, approximately 20% go on to have more serious, clinical depression. PPD may occur within 4 weeks after birth (Cuijpers, Brännmark, & van Straten, 2008) and up to a year postpartum (Beck, 2006) and can adversely impact many areas of the patient's life. Marital strain (sometimes to the point of divorce), lack of care for the infant, and, in extreme cases, suicide and infanticide are possible consequences. Research shows that there are also negative consequences for the children of affected mothers. Children are at increased risk of cognitive and motor delays. They also exhibit more emotional and behavioral problems compared with children of nondepressed mothers (Beck, 2006).

The most serious of the group of disorders classified under PPD is *postpartum psychosis*. Although episodes of postpartum psychosis often make the news, the incidence is rare: Only about 1% of new mothers develop a psychotic reaction (Vieira, 2002). Because of the severity of symptoms, it is very important that postpartum psychosis does not get confused with the more common postpartum reactions. Symptoms include delusions, hallucinations, emotional lability, and agitation; these women are very likely to be a danger to themselves and/or their baby, and immediate hospitalization is warranted (Beck, 2006).

Infertility, Reproductive Loss, and Postpartum Reactions

Women who have experienced infertility or pregnancy loss are not immune to postpartum difficulties. It seems counterintuitive that this population would be susceptible to PPD. After all, they have waited so long and worked so hard to have a baby, often putting their whole life on hold for this moment. Why is it, then, that these mothers are vulnerable to PPD?

The literature offers many possible explanations. Some of the risk factors for PPD are prenatal depression, anxiety, low self-esteem, high stress, low social support, and/or marital difficulties (Beck, 2001; Robertson, Grace, Wallington, & Stewart, 2004). It is well established that both infertile women and those who have suffered a perinatal loss undergo enormous emotional upheaval, often experiencing the exact factors listed above. When they do become pregnant, their prenatal emotional state can continue into pregnancy and postpartum.

As noted in previous sections, women may doubt the reality of their pregnancy and may feel anxious that they will incur another loss. They may be struggling with disbelief that they are normal. Their fear of suffering another loss *during pregnancy* may transfer into a fear of loss *postpartum*. Brockington et al. (2006) noted that intense fear of fetal demise was associated with a history of pregnancy loss or infertility and that, after delivery, the anxiety shifted to concerns that the baby would die. Thus, it can be surmised that the emotional state of women prior to conception can have a direct impact on them postpartum. For those who have experienced any reproductive trauma, the implications for counseling prior to conception and birth are clear. If they have psychological treatment early on, they will be better able to cope with the transition to parenthood.

Women who have had a multiple-fetal pregnancy, the likelihood of which increases with IVF and fertility-enhancing drugs, are subject to high levels of postpartum stress, depression, and anxiety. These are high-risk pregnancies and may present many more problems than singleton pregnancies. Not only are the pregnancies more difficult—often requiring long periods of bed rest— but there may be complications at birth, including an increased risk of prematurity and long hospital stays. Postpartum disorders affect more than 25% of parents of multiples (Leonard, 1998) because of the higher incidence of perinatal complications and premature births, lack of sleep, and difficulty managing the daily demands of two or more babies rather than one (Williams & Medalie, 1994).

Olshansky and Sereika (2005) put forth the hypothesis that another predictor of PPD has to do with women's "divided self." Women who had a history of infertility may present with a socially accepted outer image while internally they are experiencing rage and anger. As mentioned previously, infertile women feel less entitled to complain about parenthood because they have worked so hard and waited so long to achieve this goal. Because they have successfully conquered infertility, they deny any negative feelings about parenthood. According to relational cultural theory (Miller, 1966), the inability of these mothers to express their normal negative feelings leads to depression (Olshansky, 2003). To preserve their relationships with family and friends, these women covered up their emotions, but, paradoxically, it led them to a sense of isolation because no one was able to see what they were experiencing inside (Olshansky & Sereika, 2005). Most disturbing about this tendency is that women will not get the help they need if they are unwilling to admit their negative feelings.

Men and Postpartum

Although most of the literature on postpartum disorders focuses on women, evidence is growing that men suffer from PPD as well. Estimates of the number of men affected vary from 4% to 25% and may be attributed to hormonal changes in men during the postpartum period and/or changes in men's role as a new father (Kim & Swain, 2007). Studies have shown that there are hormonal changes in men during a partner's pregnancy and after birth. For example, higher levels of prolactin and cortisol were found in men just before the birth of their child, while their testosterone level was lower after birth (Storey, Walsh, Quinton, & Wynne-Edwards, 2000). These changes may serve a biological purpose, helping fathers attach to (Wynne-Edwards, 2001) and protect their newborn infant. More studies are needed, pre- and postbirth, to correlate changes in hormone levels with men's emotional state.

Men must adjust to their new role as fathers, with stressful demands and responsibilities that accompany newborns. Many men may not feel up to the task; they may feel incompetent and even frightened of somehow harming their baby. We often hear men lament that their "baby was so tiny, I thought I would break him." Traditionally, fathers spend less time with their infant than mothers do, perhaps because of the mother–infant bond that develops as a result of breast feeding or because of the demands of his work outside of the home. The separation and concomitant lack of practice only make fathers feel less confident in handling their baby. Men also feel jealous of the intimacy and bond between mother and child; they may feel excluded and in competition with the baby for their partner's attention (Goodman, 2002). Many men report their dissatisfaction with the lack of sexual intimacy postpartum. Condon, Boyce, and Corkindale (2004) noted a deterioration of the couple's sexual functioning from prepregnancy levels. Although men assumed that sexual activity would return to previous levels, it did not. Women's lack of interest in sex during the postpartum period can be a cause of stress in the marital relationship. These factors may all contribute to paternal PPD.

Although there is a high comorbidity between paternal and maternal PPD (Kim & Swain, 2007), there is currently no diagnosis in the *Diagnostic and Statistical Manual of Mental Disorders* (*DSM–IV*) for postpartum reactions in men. Studies of paternal PPD have used the diagnostic criteria for maternal PPD; the validity of these scales for men needs to be assessed (Kim & Swain,

2007). For women, the *DSM–IV* defines the onset of PPD as occurring within 4 weeks of delivery (American Psychiatric Association, 1994), but there is evidence that men's PPD may increase gradually over the course of the first year postpartum (Areias, Kumar, Barros, & Figueiredo, 1996). Further investigation into the unique attributes of men's postpartum reactions, development of assessment tools specifically designed for men, and the optimal treatment approach for men are areas that need further research.

Adoption and Postpartum

Postpartum reactions occur in adoptive mothers, as well, and are not limited to mild cases. Several examples of postpartum psychosis following an adoption can be found in the literature (Asch & Rubin, 1974; Van Putten & LaWall, 1981). The fact that these reactions occur in postadoptive mothers suggests that there is more than a biological or hormonal etiology at hand. The stressors of caring for a newborn—the lack of sleep, the isolation, the feelings of inadequacy as a new parent—are present whether the baby is biologically related or not. Many assume that because adoptive mothers want a baby so much, they will only have positive reactions to their child, but their responses are far more complex.

Gair (1999) found that about one third of the adoptive mothers she studied scored above the cutoff point on the Edinburgh Postnatal Depression Scale (Cox, 1986), indicating that these mothers were either at risk of or were suffering from depression and anxiety. Several factors were noted that lead to an adoptive mother's postpartum reactions: the infant's temperament (i.e., a colicky, screaming, or unsettled baby), the lack of available support, the shift in identity from working woman to motherhood, the loss of time and intimacy with her partner, and her own perception and high expectations that she needed to be a perfect mother. Just as biological mothers must reckon with the reality versus the fantasy of their newborn, and their deidealization of themselves as a parent, so must adoptive parents.

Additionally, most adoptive mothers (and fathers) have suffered through the trauma of infertility; like other new postinfertility parents, they begin their new roles already feeling inadequate because they have not been able to accomplish the basic function of bearing a child (Asch & Rubin, 1974). Not only have these parents lost control over their own fertility, they often also feel a lack of control in the adoption arrangements. Adoptive parents must pass several hurdles in order to be successful: They must "sell" themselves as suitable, must deal with the stigma of adoption—for themselves as well as for their adopted child or children, and may worry that their child will suffer damage because he or she has been relinquished. Many also have anxiety that the child will not bond with them and will have a lifelong desire to return to their biological parents. Although these fears are usually unfounded in reality, they intensify the experience of adoptive parents and add to the adjustments they must make after their baby arrives.

Unfortunately, postpartum disturbances in adoptive mothers often go undetected. One woman, whose adopted daughter is now in her 20s, had gone to her pediatrician, her primary care physician, a psychologist, and a psychiatrist in her efforts to get help after her daughter was brought home. No one put it together that she was suffering from a postpartum reaction. It was so validating to her to at last be able to identify and label what she had been going through—even 20 years after the fact.

TREATMENT OF POSTPARTUM DEPRESSION

PPD is often not acknowledged: Many women feel ashamed of their negative feelings about their child and themselves as a parent and therefore do not bring it up with their physicians. As noted earlier, this may be especially true for women who have experienced infertility or other reproductive trauma, as well as for men and adoptive parents. Although, in some cases, untreated PPD will spontaneously abate after 4 to 6 months (O'Hara, 1997), the potential risks to mother and child are too great to ignore.

Treatment for PPD typically requires a multimodal approach. Often, a combination of psychotherapy, medication, and peer support groups is the most effective. Educating patients about what they are experiencing and validating it as a reproductive trauma can do much to alleviate their shame and guilt. Support groups, led by facilitators, can be especially helpful in demonstrating to patients that they are not the only ones in the world who experience these reactions.

Women, especially those who are breast-feeding, may have resistance to pharmaceutical interventions. They fear they will harm their baby by exposing him or her to antidepressants (Appelby, Warner, Whitton, & Faragher, 1997). Some women will shorten the amount of time they had originally hoped to breast-feed in order to begin medications, but this loss may also add to their depression. A recent meta-analysis of treatments of PPD found that although pharmacological treatments may have a higher effect size, psychological interventions are also effective (Cuijpers, Brännmark, & van Straten, 2008). The authors also analyzed various psychological interventions for PPD, including cognitive behavioral therapy, interpersonal psychotherapy, counseling, and peer support. Interestingly, they found that all of the psychological modalities were about equally effective. It may be that a combination of treatments based on the severity of the PPD—utilizing medication, psychotherapy, and support—would provide the best care for these patients.

SUMMARY

The transition to parenthood is a huge adjustment for all new parents. The expectations that new parents have about their newborn and themselves are often out of proportion with the demands of caring for an infant. This may be even more difficult after the long struggle with infertility and/or perinatal loss, when so much has been invested in creating a family. Because the likelihood of depression and anxiety disorders is higher in pregnancy and parenthood following a reproductive trauma, early psychological intervention can be extremely helpful.

EPILOGUE: REWRITING
THE REPRODUCTIVE STORY

Therapeutic work with reproductive patients is an especially gratifying endeavor. These are clients with many strengths, who have had a traumatic experience in their lives. They are suffering a unique kind of pain, deriving from the largely disenfranchised losses caused by infertility, perinatal loss, complicated births, or postpartum difficulties. It is very heartening to observe the resilience of so many of these patients and their ability to use the therapeutic interventions that mental health practitioners can offer them. They respond very well to having their experiences validated as traumatic, to having their feelings normalized, to reassurance that there is no right or wrong way to process their experience—to being understood. The sense of connection they feel in the therapeutic relationship can temper their loneliness and isolation, and the therapist's nonjudgmental neutrality can help defuse their shame and guilt.

Patients readily grasp the concept of the reproductive story. It allows them to understand why they feel as they do, and it helps them to view their reproductive trauma in the broader context of their lives. The opportunity to articulate and explore their reproductive stories and their feelings about their trauma also often opens the way to deeper understanding of other parts of themselves: their childhood conflicts and roles in their family of origin, their self-concepts as adults, their defensive and coping styles, their dreams of what they hope to contribute to the world, and the intricacies and nuances of their most intimate relationships. Reproductive clients come to therapists' offices traumatized and bereft; they feel as if they are lost in a dark cave with no light or visible exits—frightened, alone, and despairing. With support and under-standing, they begin to feel hope once again. They begin to see different ways that their stories might unfold, additional options that they had been unable to imagine before, and that a sense of well-being is attainable once again, both including and apart from their reproductive lives. They come to accept that their reproductive trauma has changed them forever, but, gradually, they also begin to recognize ways in which they have grown and matured through the process.

As one patient movingly stated, "I will never be the carefree, fun-loving girl I was before all this started. But I also realize that I wouldn't really want to be. I have gained so much self-awareness through this journey, so much more depth, that my old self seems shallow and immature in comparison. I certainly wish I had not had to go through this, but if there is ever a silver lining in the dark storms of this experience, it is that I have been witness to my own resilience and gained maturity and wisdom in the process. My partner and I have traveled a horribly rocky road at times, but at this point, we are closer than we ever were, we know each other and ourselves better than we ever did, and we are facing the future together."

GLOSSARY

Amniocentesis A diagnostic procedure in which a needle is inserted through the abdominal wall into the uterus of a pregnant woman. A small amount of amniotic fluid is retrieved for use in diagnosing certain chromosomal abnormalities.

Assisted reproductive technology (ART) Fertility treatments in which a laboratory handles eggs, sperm, or embryos to increase the possibility of pregnancy.

Baby blues A relatively mild postpartum reaction that usually resolves within 10 days after birth. Approximately 60% to 80% of women experience the blues.

Blastocyst A fertilized egg in which the outer layer develops into the placenta and the inner layer forms the embryo.

Cerclage To prevent a miscarriage because of an incompetent or weak cervix, a suture is placed at the cervical opening.

Chemical pregnancy A pregnancy that is confirmed by blood test measuring the human chorionic gonadotropin (hCG) level but does not develop.

Chorionic villlus sampling (CVS) A test, early on in the pregnancy, to detect birth defects.

Clomid The drug clomiphene, which is used to stimulate ovulation.

Closed adoption Adoption of a baby, in which the identity of the birth parents is kept secret from the adoptive parents and vice versa.

Cryopreservation The freezing and storage of cells for later use. This is used for sperm samples as well as embryo preservation.

Dilation and curettage (D&C) A surgical procedure in which the cervix is expanded and then the uterine lining is scraped; often needed following miscarriage.

Dizygotic Also known as *fraternal twins*, two separate eggs become fertilized by separate sperm.

Domestic adoption An adoption of a child within the same country as the parents.

Donor A person who provides his or her own gametes (sperm or egg) for another person's use. Donors may be known (i.e., a friend or family member) or anonymous (i.e., someone who provides the gametes without revealing their identity).

Donor eggs Eggs taken from a fertile woman, which are used to assist an infertile woman to become pregnant.

Donor embryo Embryos that have been produced by one couple and donated to impregnate another woman.

Donor insemination (DI) The procedure by which donor sperm is used to impregnate a woman.

Donor sperm Sperm from a fertile man who is not the recipient's partner.

Down syndrome A genetic disorder caused by an extra chromosome 21. The syndrome is characterized by mental retardation (from mild to severe), abnormal facial features, and other medical problems.

Ectopic pregnancy   An unviable pregnancy that develops outside of the uterus, often in the fallopian tube; often creates a medical emergency.

Embryo   The early stages of development of a fertilized egg.

Endometrial biopsy   A procedure in which a small sample of the lining of the uterus (endometrium) is removed and examined to assess the health of the lining and/or to see if it can reach the appropriate stage for implantation.

Endometriosis   A condition whereby endometrial tissue grows in places other than the uterus—such as the ovaries, fallopian tubes, or the abdominal cavity. It is often associated with infertility and can cause severe pain.

Fallopian tubes   A pair of slender tubes attached to each side of the uterus. The egg travels from the ovary through the fallopian tube to the uterus. It is within the fallopian tube that fertilization of the egg by the sperm normally takes place.

Fetus   The developing baby; differentiated from the embryo, which is the early stage of development of the fertilized egg, the fetus designates the later stages, from the end of the 8th week after conception until birth.

Follicle   A sac in the ovary containing a maturing egg.

Follicle-stimulating hormone (FSH)   A pituitary hormone that promotes the growth of eggs in the ovaries in women and the formation of sperm in the testes of men. It is the hormone used in injectable ovulation drugs to stimulate production of the ovarian follicles.

Gamete   A reproductive cell whose nucleus can unite with another cell to form a new organism. In humans these are the egg and sperm cells.

Gamete intrafallopian transfer (GIFT)   A fertility procedure in which eggs are surgically removed from the ovary, combined with sperm, and then inserted into a woman's fallopian tube with the hope that fertilization will occur.

Human chorionic gonadotropin (hCG)   The hormone produced by the placenta in early pregnancy. Most pregnancy tests are based on the detection of hCG in either urine or blood samples.

Hysterectomy   A surgical procedure to remove the uterus.

Hysterosalpingogram   A diagnostic X-ray procedure to examine the shape of the uterus and look for blockage in the fallopian tubes. This is accomplished by injecting dye into the uterine cavity.

Hysteroscopy   A procedure in which a hysteroscope (a telescope-like instrument) is inserted into the uterine cavity. It is used for diagnostic as well as surgical purposes.

Implantation   The attachment of the embryo to the uterine lining in early pregnancy.

Infertility   The failure to conceive or carry a pregnancy to term after 12 months of unprotected intercourse. Primary infertility applies to those who have never had children, whereas secondary infertility describes those who have had a child but cannot conceive again.

Insemination   A procedure in which sperm is manually injected into the vagina to aid conception.

International adoption　The adoption of a child from a country different from the adoptive parents.

Intracytoplasmic sperm injection (ICSI)　A medical procedure in which sperm is injected directly into the egg.

Intrauterine insemination (IUI)　A procedure by which sperm are placed directly into the uterus (bypassing the cervix) to increase the odds of fertilization.

In vitro fertilization (IVF)　A procedure of fertilizing an egg, outside of the woman's body, in a laboratory dish. After a period of 3 to 5 days, the resulting embryo or embryos are transferred back into the woman's uterus, bypassing the fallopian tubes.

Laparoscopy　A surgical procedure in which a laparoscope (a slender, tubular instrument) is inserted through the abdomen to view, diagnose, and treat the pelvic organs.

Miscarriage　Also known as *spontaneous abortion*, the naturally occurring expulsion of the fetus before it is viable.

Monozygotic　Also known as *identical twins*, the process by which one egg fertilized by one sperm splits into two embryos with identical DNA.

Multifetal pregnancy reduction (MFPR)　Also known as *selective reduction*, a procedure used to reduce the number of fetuses in women who are pregnant with multiples.

Myomectomy　Surgery to remove fibroids (or myomas) from the uterus.

Oocyte　A cell that develops into an egg.

Open adoption　An adoption in which the identities of the birth parents and the adoptive parents are known; many times there is an ongoing relationship between both parties as the child matures.

Ovarian hyperstimulation　A painful side effect of ovarian-stimulating medications, causing the ovaries to enlarge.

Ovarian reserve　The quantity and quality of eggs remaining in a woman's ovaries.

Ovulation　The release of a mature egg from the ovary, usually occurring midway (about day 14) through a woman's menstrual cycle.

Ovulation kits　Commercially available kits that help in the prediction of ovulation in a woman's menstrual cycle.

Prenatal　Occurring prior to birth.

Perinatal　Relating to the period around birth, usually from 5 months before to 1 month after birth.

Perinatologist　An obstetrician specializing in high-risk pregnancies.

Placenta　The organ that provides nutrients to the fetus through the umbilical cord.

Polycystic ovarian syndrome (PCOS)　A condition in which there are chronic problems with ovulation, because there are many poorly developed follicles in the ovaries; other symptoms can include obesity, excess body hair, and depression.

Postcoital test (PCT)　A test that checks the quality of a woman's cervical mucus after intercourse. It looks to see whether sperm are present and moving normally.

Postpartum depression   Occurs anytime from 4 weeks to 1 year after birth. Symptoms include mood disorder, anxiety, marital strain, poor infant care, and rarely suicide or infanticide.

Postpartum psychosis   A rare (1% of new mothers) and dangerous disorder with symptoms that may include delusions, hallucinations, emotional lability, and agitation. Suicide or infanticide is possible.

Preeclampsia   Also known as *toxemia*, a condition of high blood pressure during pregnancy, which can restrict blood flow to the placenta; most often occurs in first pregnancies.

Preimplantation genetic diagnosis (PGD)   A technique used to identify genetic defects in embryos created from IVF. One or two cells of the embryo are removed and then tested for chromosomal abnormalities.

Premature birth   A birth that occurs prior to 37 weeks gestation; not uncommon with multiples.

Salpingectomy   Surgical removal of the fallopian tube.

Semen   The whitish fluid of the male ejaculate containing sperm.

Semen analysis   Tests a man's ejaculate to determine volume, number, shape, and movement of sperm.

Sperm   The male reproductive cell.

Sperm aspiration   A procedure used to obtain sperm from the male reproductive tract.

Sperm count   The number of sperm in the ejaculate.

Sperm morphology   The shape of individual sperm.

Sperm motility   The percentage of sperm that are moving in a semen sample; 50% or more should be moving rapidly.

Sperm penetration assay   A test to determine whether a man's sperm is able to fertilize eggs. This is done with specially treated hamster eggs.

Sperm washing   A procedure to separate the healthiest sperm from the seminal fluid, to increase the chance of fertilization via ART procedures.

Surrogacy   An arrangement in which one woman carries and gives birth to a child for another woman. Surrogacy can be gestational, whereby the surrogate's own genetic material is not used, or traditional, in which the surrogate's gametes are used.

Turner syndrome   A condition that affects females, in which one X chromosome is missing. It is associated with physical abnormalities as well as infertility.

Unexplained infertility   Infertility in either male or female, for which no diagnosis can be found; considered by some to be the most difficult type to cope with.

Varicocele   A varicose (or swollen) condition of the veins of the scrotum, which can cause infertility in some men; can often be corrected surgically.

Zygote   The cell formed by the union of two gametes before cell division begins.

Zygote intrafallopian transfer (ZIFT)   A procedure in which egg cells are removed from the woman and fertilized in the laboratory. The zygote, prior to cell division, is then placed in the fallopian tube.

REFERENCES

Abbey, A., Andrews, F. M., & Halman, L. J. (1994). Infertility and parenthood: Does becoming a parent increase well-being? *Journal of Consulting and Clinical Psychology*, *62*, 398–403. doi:10.1037/0022-006X.62.2.398

Allison, S., Kalucy, R., Gilchrist, P., & Jones, W. (1988). Weight preoccupation among infertile women. *International Journal of Eating Disorders*, *7*, 743–748. doi:10.1002/1098-108X(198811)7:6<743::AID-EAT2260070603>3.0.CO;2-V

American College of Obstetrics and Gynecology (ACOG). (2004). ACOG practice bulletin. Clinical management guidelines for obstetrician-gynecologists. Multiple gestation: Complicated twin, triple and high-order multifetal pregnancy. *Obstetrics and Gynecology*, *104*, 869–883.

American Counseling Association. (2005). *ACA code of ethics*. Alexandria, VA.

American Psychiatric Association. (1994). *Diagnostic and statistical manual of mental disorders* (4th ed.). Washington, DC: Author.

American Psychological Association. (2002). Ethical principles of psychologists and code of conduct. *American Psychologist*, *57*, 1060–1073. Retrieved from http://www.apa.org/ethics/code2002.html

American Psychological Association. (2005). *APA briefing paper on the impact of abortion on women*. Retrieved from http://www.apa.org/ppo/issues/womenabortfacts.html

American Society for Reproductive Medicine. (1996). *Mental health professional group bibliography*. Birmingham, AL: Author.

American Society for Reproductive Medicine. (1996–2009). *Frequently asked questions about infertility*. Retrieved from http://www.asrm.org/Patients/faqs.html

American Society for Reproductive Medicine. (2009). Guidelines on number of embryos transferred. *Fertility and Sterility*, *92*, 1518–1519. doi:10.1016/j.fertnstert.2009.08.059

American Society for Reproductive Medicine Ethics Committee. (1999). Sex selection and preimplantation genetic diagnosis. *Fertility and Sterility*, *72*, 595–598. doi:10.1016/S0015-0282(99)00319-2

American Society for Reproductive Medicine Ethics Committee. (2001). Preconception gender selection for nonmedical reasons. *Fertility and Sterility*, *75*, 861–864. doi:10.1016/S0015-0282(01)01756-3

American Society for Reproductive Medicine Ethics Committee. (2004a). Disposition of abandoned embryos. *Fertility and Sterility*, *82*(Suppl. 1), S253.

American Society for Reproductive Medicine Ethics Committee. (2004b). Informing offspring of their conception by gamete donation. *Fertility and Sterility*, *81*, 527–531. doi:10.1016/j.fertnstert.2003.11.011

Anderson, B. J., & Rosenthal, L. (2007). Acupuncture and IVF controversies (Letter to the editor). *Fertility and Sterility*, *87*, 1000.

Andrews, F. M., Abbey, A., & Halman, J. (1991). Stress from infertility, marriage factors, and subjective well-being of wives and husbands. *Journal of Health and Social Behavior, 32,* 238–253. doi:10.2307/2136806

Andrews, L. B. (1984). *New conceptions.* New York, NY: St. Martin's Press.

Anonymous. (2007). The impact that changed my life. *Professional Psychology, Research and Practice, 38,* 561–570. doi:10.1037/0735-7028.38.6.561

Antsaklis, A., Souka, A. P., Daskalakis, G., Papantoniou, N., Koutra, P., Kavalakis, Y., & Mesogitis, S. (2004). Pregnancy outcome after multifetal pregnancy reduction. *The Journal of Maternal-Fetal & Neonatal Medicine, 16,* 27–31. doi:10.1080/14767050410001728962

Appleby, L., Warner, R., Whitton, A., & Faragher, B. (1997). A controlled study of fluoxetine and cognitive-behavioral counselling in the treatment of postnatal depression. *British Medical Journal, 314,* 932–936.

Applegarth, L. D. (2000). Individual counseling and psychotherapy. In: L. H. Burns, & S. N. Covington (Eds.), *Infertility counseling: A comprehensive handbook for clinicians* (pp. 85–101). New York, NY: The Parthenon Publishing Group.

Archer, J. (1999). *The nature of grief: The evolution and psychology of reactions to loss.* Florence, KY: Taylor & Frances/Routledge.

Areias, M. E. G., Kumar, R., Barros, H., & Figueiredo, E. (1996). Correlates of postnatal depression in mothers and fathers. *The British Journal of Psychiatry, 169,* 36–41. doi:10.1192/bjp.169.1.36

Armour, K. L., & Callister, L. C. (2005). Prevention of triplets and higher order multiples. *The Journal of Perinatal & Neonatal Nursing, 19,* 103–111.

Armstrong, D. (2001). Exploring fathers' experiences of pregnancy after a prior perinatal loss. MCN, *The American Journal of Maternal/Child Nursing, 26,* 147–153. doi:10.1097/00005721-200105000-00012

Arnett, J. J. (2000). Emerging adulthood. *American Psychologist, 55,* 469–480. doi:10.1037/0003-066X.55.5.469

Arnold, J. H., & Gemma, P. B. (1994). *A child dies: A portrait of family grief.* Philadelphia, PA: The Charles Press Publishers.

Asch, S. S., & Rubin, L. J. (1974). Postpartum reactions: Some unrecognized variations. *The American Journal of Psychiatry, 131,* 870–874.

Bailey, J., Bobrow, D., Wolfe, M., & Mikach, S. (1995). Sexual orientation of adult sons of gay fathers. *Journal of Homosexuality, 31,* 124–129.

Ballou, J. (1978). The significance of reconciliative themes in the psychology of pregnancy. *Bulletin of the Menninger Clinic, 42,* 383–413.

Barlow, S. H., Burlingame, G. M., & Fuhriman, A. (2000). Therapeutic application of groups: From Pratt's "thought control classes" to modern group psychotherapy. *Group Dynamics, 4,* 115–134. doi:10.1037/1089-2699.4.1.115

Barrett, M. S., & Berman, J. S. (2001). Is psychotherapy more effective when therapists disclose information about themselves? *Journal of Consulting and Clinical Psychology, 69,* 597–603. doi:10.1037/0022-006X.69.4.597

Bartlett, J. A. (1991). Psychiatric issues in non-anonymous oocyte donation. Motivations and expectations of women donors and recipients. *Psychosomatics, 32*, 433–437.

Bartlik, B., Greene, K., Graf, M., Sharma, G., & Melnick, H. (1997). Examining PTSD as a complication of infertility. *Medscape Womens Health, 2*, 1. Retrieved from http://www.ncbi.nlm.nih.gov/pubmed/9746683

Beaurepaire, J., Jones, M., Thiering, P., Saunders, D., & Tennant, C. (1994). Psychosocial adjustment to infertility and its treatment: Male and female responses at different stages of IVF/ET treatment. *Journal of Psychosomatic Research, 38*, 229–240. doi:10.1016/0022-3999(94)90118-X

Beck, C. T. (2001). Predictors of postpartum depression: An update. *Nursing Research, 50*, 275–285. doi:10.1097/00006199-200109000-00004

Beck, C. T. (2006). Postpartum depression: It isn't just the blues. *The American Journal of Nursing, 106*, 40–50.

Becker, G., Butler, A., & Nachtigall, R. D. (2005). Resemblance talk: A challenge for parents whose children were conceived with donor gametes in the US. *Social Science & Medicine, 61*, 1300–1309. doi:10.1016/j.socscimed.2005.01.018

Benedek, T. (1952). Infertility as a psychosomatic defense. *Fertility and Sterility, 3*, 527–541.

Benedek, T. (1959). Parenthood as a developmental phase. *Journal of the American Psychoanalytic Association, 7*, 389–417. doi:10.1177/000306515900700301

Benedek, T. (1970). The psychobiology of pregnancy. In E. J. Anthon and T. Benedek (Eds.), *Parenthood: Its psychology and psychopathology* (pp. 137–155). Boston, MA: Little, Brown & Co.

Bennett, S. M., Litz, B. T., Lee, B. S., & Maguen, S. (2005). The scope and impact of perinatal loss: Current status and future directions. *Professional Psychology, Research and Practice, 36*, 180–187. doi:10.1037/0735-7028.36.2.180

Berg, B. J., & Wilson, J. F. (1991). Psychological functioning across stages of treatment for infertility. *Journal of Behavioral Medicine, 14*, 11–26. doi:10.1007/BF00844765

Berg, B. J., Wilson, J. F., & Weingartner, P. J. (1991). Psychological sequelae of infertility treatment: The role of gender and sex-role identification. *Social Science & Medicine, 33*, 1071–1080. doi:10.1016/0277-9536(91)90012-2

Bernstein, J., Potts, N., & Mattox, J. H. (1985). Assessment of psychological dysfunction associated with infertility. *Journal of Obstetric, Gynecologic, and Neonatal Nursing, 14*(Suppl.), 63s–66s. doi:10.1111/j.1552-6909.1985.tb02803.x

Bibring, G. (1959). Some consideration of the psychological processes in pregnancy. *The Psychoanalytic Study of the Child, 14*, 113–121.

Blenner, J. L. (1992). Stress and mediators: Patients' perceptions of infertility treatment. *Nursing Research, 41*, 92–97.

Bloom, K., Delmore-Ko, P., Masataka, N., & Carli, L. (1999). Possible self as parent in Canadian, Italian, and Japanese young adults. *Canadian Journal of Behavioural Science, 31*, 198–207. doi:10.1037/h0087088

Bloomgarden, A., & Mennuti, R. B. (2009). Therapist self-disclosure: Beyond the taboo. In A. Bloomgarden & R. B. Mennuti (Eds.), *Psychotherapist revealed* (pp. 3–15). New York, NY: Routledge.

Blos, P. (1962). *On adolescence.* New York, NY: Free Press.

Blos, P. (1967). The second individuation process of adolescence. *The Psychoanalytic Study of the Child, 22,* 162–186.

Boivin, J. (2003). A review of psychosocial interventions in infertility. *Social Science & Medicine, 57,* 2325–2341. doi:10.1016/S0277-9536(03)00138-2

Borders, L. D., Black, L. K., & Pasley, B. K. (1998). Are adopted children and their parents at greater risk for negative outcomes? *Family Relations, 47,* 237–241. doi:10.2307/584972

Born, L., Phillips, S. D., Steiner, M. & Soares, C. N. (2005). Trauma & the reproductive lifecycle in women. *Revista Brasileira de Psiquiatria, 27*(Suppl. 2), S65–S72.

Born, L., Soares, C. N., Phillips, S. D., Jung, M., & Steiner, M. (2006). Women and reproductive-related trauma. *Annals of the New York Academy of Sciences, 1071,* 491–494. doi:10.1196/annals.1364.049

Bowlby, J. (1969). *Attachment, separation and loss.* New York, NY: Basic Books.

Boxer, A. (1996). Infertility and sexual dysfunction. *Infertility and Reproductive Medicine Clinics, 7,* 565–575.

Boyd-Bragadeste, K. L. (1998). *A biopsychosocial approach to understanding postpartum adjustment* (Doctoral dissertation). California School of Professional Psychology, San Diego, CA.

Britt, D. W., & Evans, M. I. (2007a). Information-sharing among couples considering multifetal pregnancy reduction. *Fertility and Sterility, 87,* 490–495.

Britt, D. W., & Evans, M. I. (2007b). Sometimes doing the right thing sucks: Frame combinations and multi-fetal pregnancy reduction decision difficulty. *Social Science & Medicine, 65,* 2342–2356. doi:10.1016/j.socscimed.2007.06.026

Brockington, I. F., Macdonald, E., & Wainscott, G. (2006). Anxiety, obsessions and morbid preoccupations in pregnancy and the puerperium. *Archives of Women's Mental Health, 9,* 253–263. doi:10.1007/s00737-006-0134-z

Brownlee, K., & Oikonen, J. (2004). Toward a theoretical framework for perinatal bereavement. *British Journal of Social Work, 34,* 517–529. doi:10.1093/bjsw/bch063

Bryan, E. M. (1995). The death of a twin. *Palliative Medicine, 9,* 187–192. doi:10.1177/026921639500900303

Bryan, E. M. (2002). Loss in higher multiple pregnancy and multifetal pregnancy reduction. *Twin Research, 5,* 169–174. doi:10.1375/136905202320227826

Bryan, E. M., & Hallett, F. (1997). *Bereavement: guidelines for professionals.* London, England: Multiple Births Foundation.

Bryan, E. M., & Higgins, R. (2002). Introduction. *Twin Research: The Official Journal of the International Society for Twin Studies, 5,* 146–148.

Bullough, V. L. (2004). Artificial insemination. *glbtq: An encyclopedia of gay, lesbian, bisexual, transgender, and queer culture*. Retrieved from http://www.glbtq.com/social-sciences/artificial_insemination.html.

Burns, L. H. (2000). Sexual counseling and infertility. In L. H. Burns & S. N. Covington (Eds.), *Infertility counseling: A comprehensive handbook for clinicians* (pp. 149–176). New York, NY: The Parthenon Publishing Group.

Burns, L. H., & Covington, S. N. (2000). Psychology of infertility. In L. H. Burns, & S. N. Covington, (Eds.), *Infertility counseling: A comprehensive handbook for clinicians* (pp. 3–25). New York, NY: The Parthenon Publishing Group.

Butler, R. R., & Koraleski, S. (1990). Infertility: A crisis with no resolution. *Journal of Mental Health Counseling, 12*, 151–163.

Cain, A., & Cain, B. (1964). On replacing a child. *Journal of the American Academy of Child Psychiatry, 3*, 443–456. doi:10.1016/S0002-7138(09)60158-8

Campbell, E. (1986). *The childless marriage: An exploratory study of couples who do not want children*. New York, NY: Tavistock.

Capitulo, K. L. (2004). Perinatal grief online. *MCN, The American Journal of Maternal/Child Nursing, 29*, 305–311. doi:10.1097/00005721-200409000-00008

Capitulo, K. L. (2005). Evidence for healing interventions with perinatal bereavement. *MCN, The American Journal of Maternal/Child Nursing, 30*, 389–396. doi:10.1097/00005721-200511000-00007

Centers for Disease Control and Prevention. (2002). Use of assisted reproductive technology—United States, 1996 and 1998. *MMWR Weekly, 51*(5), 97–101.

Chabot, J. M., & Ames, B. D. (2004). "It wasn't 'let's get pregnant and go do it'": Decision making in lesbian couples planning motherhood via donor insemination. *Family Relations, 53*, 348–356. doi:10.1111/j.0197-6664.2004.00041.x

Chan, C. H. Y., Ng, E. H. Y., Chan, C. L. W., Ho, P. C., & Chan, T. H. Y. (2006). Effectiveness of psychosocial group intervention for reducing anxiety in women undergoing in vitro fertilization: a randomized controlled study. *Fertility and Sterility, 85*, 339–346. doi:10.1016/j.fertnstert.2005.07.1310

Chavarro, J. E., Rich-Edwards, J. W., Rosner, B. A., & Willett, W. C. (2007). Diet and lifestyle in the prevention of ovulatory disorder infertility. *Obstetrics and Gynecology, 110*, 1050–1058.

Chavarro, J. E., Rich-Edwards, J. W., Rosner, B. A., & Willett, W. C. (2008). Use of multivitamins, intake of B vitamins, and risk of ovulatory infertility. *Fertility and Sterility, 89*, 668–676. doi:10.1016/j.fertnstert.2007.03.089

Child, T. J., Henderson, A. M., & Tan, S. L. (2004). The desire for multiple pregnancy in male and female infertility patients. *Human Reproduction, 19*, 558–561. doi:10.1093/humrep/deh097

Colarusso, C. A. (1990). The third individuation: The effect of biological parenthood on separation-individuation processes in adulthood. *The Psychoanalytic Study of the Child, 45*, 179–194.

Colarusso, C. A., & Nemiroff, R. A. (1987). Clinical implications of adult developmental theory. *The American Journal of Psychiatry, 144*, 1263–1270.

Collins, J. (2006). The play of chance. *Fertility and Sterility, 85*, 1364–1367. doi:10.1016/j.fertnstert.2005.10.064

Collopy, K. S. (2004). "I couldn't think that far": Infertile women's decision making about multifetal reduction. *Research in Nursing & Health, 27*, 75–86. doi:10.1002/nur.20012

Comstock, D. L. (2009). Confronting life's adversities: Self-disclosure in print and in session. In A. Bloomgarden & R. B. Mennuti (Eds.), *Psychotherapist revealed* (pp. 257–273). New York, NY: Routledge.

Condon, J. T., Boyce, P., & Corkindale, C. J. (2004). The first-time fathers study: A prospective study of the mental health and wellbeing of men during the transition to parenthood. *The Australian and New Zealand Journal of Psychiatry, 38*(1–2), 56–64. doi:10.1111/j.1440-1614.2004.01298.x

Conway, P., & Valentine, D. (1987). Reproductive losses and grieving. *Journal of Social Work & Human Sexuality, 6*, 43–64.

Cornell, W. F. (2007). The intricate intimacies of psychotherapy and questions of self-disclosure. *European Journal of Psychotherapy and Counselling, 9*, 51–61. doi:10.1080/13642530601164372

Côté-Arsenault, D. (2003). Weaving babies lost in pregnancy into the fabric of the family. *Journal of Family Nursing, 9*, 23–37. doi:10.1177/1074840702239489

Cousineau, T. M., Green, T. C., Corsini, E., Seibring, A., Showstack, M. F., Applegarth, L., . . . Perloe, M. (2008). Online psychoeducational support for infertile women: A randomized controlled trial. *Human Reproduction, 23*, 554–566. doi:10.1093/humrep/dem306

Covington, S. N. (2006). Group approaches to infertility counseling. In S. N. Covington & L. H. Burns (Eds.), *Infertility counseling: A comprehensive handbook for clinicians* (2nd ed., pp. 156–168). New York, NY: Cambridge University Press.

Cowan, C. P., Cowan, P. A., Heming, G., Garrett, E., Coysh, W. S., Curtis-Boles, H., & Boles, A. J. (1985). Transitions to parenthood: His, hers, and theirs. *Journal of Family Issues, 6*, 451–481. doi:10.1177/019251385006004004

Cox, J. (1986). *Postnatal depression: A guide for health professionals*. Edinburgh, Scotland: Churchill Livingstone.

Craig, L. B., Criniti, A. R., Hansen, K. R., Marshall, L. A., & Soules, M. R. (2007). Acupuncture lowers pregnancy rates when performed before and after embryo transfer. *Fertility and Sterility, 88*(Suppl. 1), S40. doi:10.1016/j.fertnstert.2007.07.143

Crawford, I., McLeod, A., Zamboni, B. D., & Jordan, M. B. (1999). Psychologists' attitudes toward gay and lesbian parenting. *Professional Psychology, Research and Practice, 30*, 394–401. doi:10.1037/0735-7028.30.4.394

Cudmore, L. (2005). Becoming parents in the contest of loss. *Sexual and Relationship Therapy, 20*, 299–308. doi:10.1080/14681990500141204

Cuijpers, P., Brännmark, J. G., & van Straten, A. (2008). Psychological treatment of postpartum depression: A meta-analysis. *Journal of Clinical Psychology, 64,* 103–118. doi:10.1002/jclp.20432

Czeizel, A. E. & Dudas, I. (1992). Prevention of the first occurrence of neural-tube defects by periconceptional vitamin supplementation. *New England Journal of Medicine, 327,* 1832–1835.

Daniels, K. (1993). Infertility counselling: The need for a psychosocial perspective. *British Journal of Social Work, 23,* 501–515. doi:10.1093/bjsw/23.5.501

Daniluk, J. C. (1991). Strategies for counseling infertile couples. *Journal of Counseling and Development, 69,* 317–320.

Daniluk, J. C. (2001). "If we had it to do over again . . .": Couples' reflections on their experiences of infertility treatments. *The Family Journal, 9,* 122–133. doi:10.1177/1066480701092006

Daniluk, J. C., & Hurtig-Mitchell, J. (2003). Themes of hope and healing: Infertile couples' experiences of adoption. *Journal of Counseling and Development, 81,* 389–399.

Daniluk, J. C., & Tench, E. (2007). Long-term adjustment of infertile couples following unsuccessful medical intervention. *Journal of Counseling and Development, 85,* 89–100.

Daly, K. (1989). Anger among prospective adoptive parents: Structural determinants and management strategies. *Clinical Sociology Review, 7,* 80–96.

DeFrain, J. (1991). Learning about grief from normal families: SIDS, stillbirth, and miscarriage. *Journal of Marital and Family Therapy, 17,* 215–232. doi:10.1111/j.1752-0606.1991.tb00890.x

De Lacey, S. (2007). Decisions for the fate of frozen embryos: Fresh insights into patients' thinking and their rationales for donating or discarding embryos. *Human Reproduction, 22,* 1751–1758. doi:10.1093/humrep/dem056

De Sutter, P., Van der Elst, J., Coetsier, T., & Dhont, M. (2003). Single embryo transfer and multiple pregnancy rate reduction in IVF/ICSI: A 5-year appraisal. *Reproductive Biomedicine Online, 6,* 464–469.

Deutsch, H. (1945). *The psychology of women: Motherhood* (Vol. 2). New York, NY: Grune & Stratton.

Dhillon, R., Cumming, C. E., & Cumming, D. C. (2000). Psychological well-being and coping patterns in infertile men. *Fertility and Sterility, 74,* 702–706.

Diamond, D. J. (2005). *Psychology of reproductive trauma: A developmental perspective.* Paper presented at the American Psychological Association Annual Convention, Washington, DC.

Diamond, M. O. (1983). *The transition to adolescence in girls: Conscious and unconscious experiences of puberty* (Doctoral dissertation). University of Michigan, Ann Arbor, MI.

Diamond, M. O. (2005). *Couples and reproductive trauma: Differences between men and women.* Paper presented at the American Psychological Association Annual Convention, Washington, DC.

Dieterle, S., Ying, G., Hatzmann, W., & Neuer, A. (2006). Effect of acupuncture on the outcome of in vitro fertilization and intracytoplasmic sperm injection: A randomized, prospective, controlled clinical study. *Fertility and Sterility, 85,* 1347–1351. doi:10.1016/j.fertnstert.2005.09.062

Doka, K. J. (1989). Disenfranchised grief. In K. J. Doka (Ed.), *Disenfranchised grief: Recognizing hidden sorrow* (pp. 3–11). New York, NY: Lexington Books/Free Press.

Domar, A. D. (2006). Acupuncture and infertility: We need to stick to good science. *Fertility and Sterility, 85,* 1359–1361. doi:10.1016/j.fertnstert.2005.10.063

Domar, A. D., Broome, A., Zuttermeister, P., Seibel, M., & Friedman, R. (1992). The prevalence and predictability of depression in infertile women. *Fertility and Sterility, 6,* 1158–1163.

Domar, A. D., Clapp, D., Slawsby, E., Kessel, B., Orav, J., & Freizinger, M. (2000). The impact of group psychological interventions of distress in infertile women. *Health Psychology, 19,* 568–575. doi:10.1037/0278-6133.19.6.568

Domar, A. D., Meshay, I., Kelliher, J., Wang, S., & Alper, M. (2006). The impact of acupuncture on IVF outcome. *Fertility and Sterility, 86*(Suppl.), S378–S379. doi:10.1016/j.fertnstert.2006.07.1042

Domar, A. D., Seibel, M., & Benson, H. (1990). The mind/body program for infertility: A new behavioral treatment approach for women with infertility. *Fertility and Sterility, 53,* 246–249.

Domar, A. D., Zuttermeister, P., & Friedman, R. (1993). The psychological impact of infertility: A comparison to patients with other medical conditions. *Journal of Psychosomatic Obstetrics and Gynaecology, 14,* 45–52.

Domar, A. D., Zuttermeister, P., & Friedman, R. (1999). The relationship between distress and conception in infertile women. *Journal of the American Women's Association, 54,* 196–198.

Drescher, J., Glazer, D. F., Crespi, L., & Schwartz, D. (2005). What is a mother? Gay and lesbian perspectives on parenting. In S. F. Brown (Ed.), *What do mothers want? Developmental perspective, clinical challenges* (pp. 87–103). Hillsdale, NJ: The Analytic Press.

Dunne, G. A. (1999). *The different dimensions of gay fatherhood: Exploding the myths* [Gender Institute discussion paper]. London School of Economics Gender Institute, London, England.

Dunne, G. A. (2000). Opting into motherhood: Lesbians blurring the boundaries and transforming the meaning of parenthood and kinship. *Gender & Society, 14,* 11–35. doi:10.1177/089124300014001003

Dunson, D. B., Baird, D. D., & Columbo, B. (2004). Increased infertility with age in men and women. *Obstetrics & Gynecology, 103,* 51–56.

Egan, J. (2006, March 19). Wanted: A few good sperm. *The New York Times.* Retrieved from http://www.nytimes.com/2006/03/19/magazine/319dad.html?pagewanted= print.

Egg Donation Inc. (2008). Retrieved from http://eggdonor.com

Epstein, Y. M., Rosenberg, H. S., Grant, T. V., & Hemenway, N. (2002). Use of the Internet as the only outlet for talking about infertility. *Fertility and Sterility, 78,* 507–514. doi:10.1016/S0015-0282(02)03270-3

Erikson, E. (1963). *Childhood and Society* (2nd ed.). New York, NY: Norton.

Evans, M. I., Kaufman, M. I., Urban, A. J., Britt, D. W., & Fletcher, J. C. (2004). Fetal reduction from twins to singleton: A reasonable consideration? *American College of Obstetricians and Gynecologists, 104,* 102–109.

Fergusson, D. M., Horwood, L. J., & Ridder, E. M. (2006). Abortion in young women and subsequent mental health. *Journal of Child Psychology and Psychiatry, and Allied Disciplines, 47,* 16–24. doi:10.1111/j.1469-7610.2005.01538.x

Fisch, H. (2009). The aging male and his biological clock. *Geriatrics, 64,* 14–19.

Freeman, N. (2005). When the therapist is infertile. In A. Rosen & J. Rosen (Eds.), *Frozen dreams: Psychodynamic dimensions of infertility and assisted reproduction* (pp. 50–68). Hillsdale, NJ: The Analytic Press.

Freud, S. (2000). Recommendations to physicians practicing psycho-analysis. In *The standard edition of the psychological works of Sigmund Freud* (pp. 1–120). London, England: Hogarth Press (Original work published 1912).

Freud, S. (1953). *The interpretation of dreams.* London, England: Hogarth Press.

Friedman, C. (2007). First comes love, then comes marriage, then comes baby carriage: Perspectives on gay parenting and reproductive technology. *Journal of Infant, Child, and Adolescent Psychotherapy, 6,* 111–123. doi:10.1080/15289160701624407

Frisch, R. E. (1977). Food intake, fatness, and reproductive ability. In R. A. Vigersky (Ed.), *Anorexia nervosa* (pp. 149–161). New York, NY: Raven Press.

Furst, K. (1983). *Origins and evolution of women's dreams in early adulthood* (Unpublished doctoral dissertation). California School of Professional Psychology, Berkeley, CA.

Gair, S. (1999). Distress and depression in new motherhood: Research with adoptive mothers highlights important contributing factors. *Child & Family Social Work, 4,* 55–66. doi:10.1046/j.1365-2206.1999.00098.x

Galton, D. J. (2005). Eugenics: Some lessons from the past. *Ethics, Law and Moral Philosophy of Reproductive Biomedicine, 1,* 133–136.

Garner, C. H. (1985). Pregnancy after infertility. *Journal of Obstetric, Gynecologic, and Neonatal Nursing, 14*(Suppl.), 58s–62s. doi:10.1111/j.1552-6909.1985.tb02802.x

Geller, J. D. (2003). Self-disclosure in psychoanalytic-existential therapy. *Journal of Clinical Psychology, 59,* 541–554.

Geller, P. A. (2004). Pregnancy as a stressful life event. *CNS Spectrums, 9,* 188–197.

Gerrity, D. A. (2001). A biopsychosocial theory of infertility. *The Family Journal, 9,* 151–158. doi:10.1177/1066480701092009

Gilbert, K. R. (1996). "We've had the same loss, why don't we have the same grief?" Loss and differential grief in families. *Death Studies, 20,* 269–283. doi:10.1080/07481189608252781

Goldfried, M. R., Burckell, L. A., & Eubanks-Carter, C. (2003). Therapist self-disclosure in cognitive-behavior therapy. *Journal of Clinical Psychology, 59*, 555–568.

Goldstein, E. G. (1994). Self-disclosure in treatment: What therapists do and don't talk about. *Clinical Social Work Journal, 22*, 417–433. doi:10.1007/BF02190331

Golombok, S., Brewaeys, A., Giavazzi, M. T., Guerra, D., MacCallum, F., & Rust, J. (2002). The European study of assisted reproduction families: The transition into adolescence. *Human Reproduction, 17*, 830–840. doi:10.1093/humrep/17.3.830

Golombok, S., Lycett, E., MacCallum, F., Jadva, V., Murray, C., Rust, J., . . . Margara, R. (2004). Parenting infants conceived by gamete donation. *Journal of Family Psychology, 18*, 443–452. doi:10.1037/0893-3200.18.3.443

Golombok, S., Spencer, A., & Rutter, M. (1983). Children in lesbian and single parent households: Psychosexual and psychiatric appraisal. *Journal of Child Psychology and Psychiatry, 24*, 551–572. doi:10.1111/j.1469-7610.1983.tb00132.x

Golombok, S., & Tasker, F. (1996). Do parents influence the sexual orientation of their children? Findings from a longitudinal study of lesbian families. *Developmental Psychology, 32*, 3–11.

Goodman, J. H. (2005). Becoming an involved father of an infant. *Journal of Obstetric, Gynecologic, and Neonatal Nursing, 34*, 190–200. doi:10.1177/0884217505274581

Green, R., Mandel, J. B., Hotvedt, M. E., Gray, J., & Smith, L. (1986). Lesbian mothers and their children: A comparison with solo parent heterosexual mothers and their children. *Archives of Sexual Behavior, 15*, 167–184. doi:10.1007/BF01542224

Greenfeld, D. A., Diamond, M. P., & DeCherney, A. H. (1988). Grief reactions following in-vitro fertilization treatment. *Journal of Psychosomatic Obstetrics and Gynaecology, 8*, 169–174. doi:10.3109/01674828809016784

Greenfeld, D. A., & Klock, S. C. (2004). Disclosure decisions among known and anonymous oocyte donation recipients. *Fertility and Sterility, 81*, 1565–1571. doi:10.1016/j.fertnstert.2003.10.041

Greil, A. L., Leitko, T. A., & Porter, K. L. (1988). Infertility: His and hers. *Gender & Society, 2*, 172–199. doi:10.1177/089124388002002004

Greil, A. L., Porter, K. L., & Leitko, T. A. (1990). Sex and intimacy among infertile couples. *Journal of Psychology & Human Sexuality, 2*, 117–138. doi:10.1300/J056v02n02_08

Gruen, D. S. (1993). A group psychotherapy approach to postpartum depression. *International Journal of Group Psychotherapy, 43*, 191–203.

Gutmann, J. N., & Covington, S. N. (2006). Complementary and alternative medicine in infertility counseling. In S. N. Covington & L. H. Burns (Eds.), *Infertility counseling: A comprehensive handbook for clinicians* (2nd ed., pp. 196–211). New York, NY: Cambridge University Press.

Hadley, E., & Stuart, J. (2009). The expression of parental identifications in lesbian mothers' work and family arrangements. *Psychoanalytic Psychology, 26*, 42–68. doi:10.1037/a0014676

Haftek, J. (2008). Impact of the abortion process on male partners: An exploratory study of their conscious and unconscious experiences. *Dissertation Abstracts International: Section B. Sciences and Engineering, Volume* 69(6-B).

Hare, J., & Skinner, D. (2008). "Whose child is this?": Determining legal status for lesbian parents who used assisted reproductive technologies. *Family Relations, 57*, 365–375. doi:10.1111/j.1741-3729.2008.00506.x

Hart, V. A. (2002). Infertility and the role of psychotherapy. *Issues in Mental Health Nursing, 23*, 31–41. doi:10.1080/01612840252825464

Hassan, M. A., & Killick, S. R. (2003). Effect of male age on fertility: Evidence for the decline in male fertility with increasing age. *Fertility & Sterility, 79*(Suppl. 3), 1520–1527.

Heffner, L. J. (2004). Advanced maternal age—How old is too old? *The New England Journal of Medicine, 351*, 1927–1929. doi:10.1056/NEJMp048087

Hendrix, H. (1988). *Getting the love you want: A guide for couples.* New York, NY: Henry Holt & Company.

Hertz, R. & Ferguson, F. I. T. (1997). Kinship strategies and self-sufficiency among single mothers by choice: Post modern family ties. *Qualitative Sociology, 20*, 187–209.

Hill, C. E., & Knox, S. (2001). Self-disclosure. *Psychotherapy, 38*, 413–417. doi:10.1037/0033-3204.38.4.413

Himmel, W., Meyer, J., Kochen, M. M., & Michelmann, H. W. (2005). Information needs and visitors' experience of an Internet expert forum on infertility. *Journal of Medical Internet Research, 7*, e20. doi:10.2196/jmir.7.2.e20

Hirsch, M. B., & Mosher, W. D. (1987). Characteristics of infertile women in the United States and their use of infertility services. *Fertility and Sterility, 47*, 618–625.

Hoffman, D. I., Zellman, G. L., Fair, C. C., Mayer, J. F., Zeitz, J. G., Gibbons, W. E., & Turner, T. G. (2003). Cryopreserved embryos in the United States and their availability for research. *Fertility and Sterility, 79*, 1063–1069. doi:10.1016/S0015-0282(03)00172-9

Hoffman, I. (1992). Some practical implications of a social constructivist view of the psychoanalytic situation. *Psychoanalytic Dialogues, 2*, 287–304. doi:10.1080/10481889209538934

Hollingsworth, L. D. (2005). Ethical considerations in prenatal sex selection. *Health & Social Work, 30*, 126–134.

Hooker, K., Fiese, B. H., Jenkins, L., Morfei, M. Z., & Schwagler, J. (1996). Possible selves among parents of infants and preschoolers. *Developmental Psychology, 32*, 542–550. doi:10.1037/0012-1649.32.3.542

Hosaka, T., Matsubayashi, H., Sugiyama, Y., Izumi, S., & Makino, T. (2002). Effect of psychiatric group intervention on natural-killer cell activity and pregnancy rate. *General Hospital Psychiatry, 24,* 353–356. doi:10.1016/S0163-8343(02)00194-9

Hosaka, T., Tokuda, Y., & Sugiyama, Y. (2000). Effects of a structured psychiatric intervention on cancer patients' emotions and coping styles. *International Journal of Clinical Oncology, 5,* 188–191. doi:10.1007/PL00012036

Huang, S. T., & Chen, A. P. (2008). Traditional Chinese medicine and infertility. *Current Opinion in Obstetrics & Gynecology, 20,* 211–215. doi:10.1097/GCO. 0b013e3282f88e22

Hynie, M., & Burns, L. H. (2006). Cross-cultural issues in infertility counseling. In S. N. Covington & L. H. Burns (Eds.), *Infertility counseling: A comprehensive handbook for clinicians* (2nd ed., pp. 61–82). New York, NY: Cambridge University Press.

Ivaldi, G. (2000). *Surveying adoptions: A comprehensive analysis of local authority adoptions 1998/9.* London, England: British Association for Adoption and Fostering.

Jaffe, J., Diamond, M. O., & Diamond, D. J. (2005). *Unsung lullabies: Understanding and coping with infertility.* New York, NY: St. Martin's Press.

Jordan, C., & Revenson, T. A. (1999). Gender differences in coping with infertility: A meta-analysis. *Journal of Behavioral Medicine, 22,* 341–358. doi:10.1023/A: 1018774019232

Jordan, J. V. (2000). The role of mutual empathy in relational/cultural therapy. *Journal of Clinical Psychology, 56,* 1005–1016. doi:10.1002/1097-4679(200008)56:8<1005:: AID-JCLP2>3.0.CO;2-L

Jourard, S. M. (1971). *The transparent self.* New York, NY: Van Nostrand Reinhold.

Kim, P., & Swain, J. E. (2007). Sad dads: Paternal postpartum depression. *Psychiatry, 4,* 36–47.

Kittrell, D. (1998). A comparison of the evolution of men's and women's dreams in Daniel Levinson's theory of adult development. *Journal of Adult Development, 5,* 105–115. doi:10.1023/A:1023039611468

Klass, D. (2006). Continuing conversation about continuing bonds. *Death Studies, 30,* 843–858. doi:10.1080/07481180600886959

Klock, S. C. (2006). Psychosocial evaluation of the infertile patient. In S. N. Covington & L. H. Burns (Eds.), *Infertility counseling: A comprehensive handbook for clinicians* (2nd ed., pp. 83–96). New York, NY: Cambridge University Press.

Klock, S. C., Shenin, S., & Kazer, R. R. (2001). The disposition of unused frozen embryos. *The New England Journal of Medicine, 345,* 69–70. doi:10.1056/ NEJM200107053450118

K. M. v. E. G., 118 Cal. App. 4th 477 (Cal. 2004).

Knox, S., Hess, S., Peterson, D., & Hill, C. E. (1997). A qualitative analysis of client perceptions of the effects of helpful therapist self-disclosure in long-term therapy. *Journal of Counseling Psychology, 44,* 274–283. doi:10.1037/0022-0167.44.3.274

Knox, S., & Hill, C. E. (2003). Therapist self-disclosure: Research-based suggestions for practitioners. *Journal of Clinical Psychology, 59,* 529–539.

Kohut, H. (1977). *The Restoration of the Self*. New York, NY: International Universities Press.

Korenromp, M. J., Page-Christiaens, G. C. M. L., van den Bout, J., Mulder, E. J. H., & Visser, G. H. A. (2007). Maternal decision to terminate pregnancy after a diagnosis of Down syndrome. *American Journal of Obstetrics & Gynecology, 196*, 149.e1–149.e11.

Kristine H. v. Lisa R., 120 App. 4th 143 (Cal. 2004).

Kroth, J., Garcia, M., Hallgren, M., LeGrue, E., Ross, L. M., & Scalise, J. (2004). Perinatal loss, trauma, and dream reports. *Psychological Reports, 94*(3, Pt. 1), 877–882. doi:10.2466/PR0.94.3.877-882

Kubler-Ross, E. (1969). *On death and dying*. New York, NY: Macmillan.

La Joie, M. (2003). *Psychological adjustment of women experiencing secondary infertility* (Unpublished doctoral dissertation). New York University, New York, NY.

Lambda Legal. (2008). *Overview of state adoption laws*. Retrieved from http://www.lambdalegal.org/our-work/issues/marriage-relationships-family/parenting/overview-of-state-adoption.html.

Lane, R. C., & Hull, J. W. (1990). Self-disclosure and classical psychoanalysis. In G. Stricker & M. Fischer (Eds.), *Self-disclosure in the therapeutic relationship* (pp. 31–46). New York, NY: Plenum Press.

Lasker, J. N., & Toedter, L. J. (2000). Predicting outcomes after pregnancy loss: Results from studies using the Perinatal Grief Scale. *Illness, Crisis & Loss, 8*, 350–372.

Lazarus, R. S., & Folkman, S. (1984). *Stress, appraisal, and coping*. New York, NY: Springer.

Lee, T. Y., Sun, G. H., & Chao, S. C. (2001). The effect of an infertility diagnosis on the distress, marital and sexual satisfaction between husbands and wives in Taiwan. *Human Reproduction, 16*, 1762–1767. doi:10.1093/humrep/16.8.1762

Lentner, E., & Glazer, G. (1991). Infertile couples perceptions of infertility support-group participation. *Health Care for Women International, 12*, 317–330. doi:10.1080/07399339109515954

Leon, I. G. (1990). *When a baby dies*. New Haven, CT: Yale University Press.

Leon, I. G. (1996). Reproductive loss: Barriers to psychoanalytic treatment. *The Journal of the American Academy of Psychoanalysis, 24*, 341–352.

Leonard, L. (1998). Depression and anxiety disorder during multiple pregnancy and parenthood. *Journal of Obstetric, Gynecologic, and Neonatal Nursing, 27*, 329–337. doi:10.1111/j.1552-6909.1998.tb02656.x

Leventhal, A. M. (2008). Sadness, depression and avoidance behavior. *Behavior Modification, 32*, 759–779.

Levinson, D. J. (1978). *The seasons of a man's life*. New York, NY: Alfred Knopf.

Levinson, D. J. (1986). A conception of adult development. *American Psychologist, 41*, 3–13.

Levinson, D. J. (1996). *The seasons of a woman's life*. New York, NY: Alfred Knopf.

Levy-Shiff, R., Bar, O., & Har-Even, D. (1990). Psychological adjustment of adoptive parents-to-be. *American Journal of Orthopsychiatry, 60*, 258–267. doi:10.1037/h0079165

Lewin, T. (2007, May 22). Out of grief grows an advocacy for legal certificate of stillborn birth. *The New York Times*, p. A16.

Lindemann, E. (1944). Symptomatology and management of acute grief. *The American Journal of Psychiatry, 101*, 141–148.

Lobaugh, E. R., Clements, P. T., Averill, J. B., & Olguin, D. L. (2006). Gay-male couples who adopt: Challenging historical and contemporary social trends toward becoming a family. *Perspectives in Psychiatric Care, 42*, 184–195. doi:10.1111/j.1744-6163.2006.00081.x

Lutjen, P., Travinson, A., Lecton, J., Findlay, J., Wood, C., & Renou, P. (1984, January 12). The establishment and maintenance of pregnancy using IVF and embryo donation in a patient with primary ovarian failure. *Nature, 307*, 174–175. doi:10.1038/307174a0

Lycett, E., Daniels, K., Curson, R., Chir, B., & Golombok, S. (2004). Offspring created as a result of donor insemination: A study of family relationships, child adjustment, and disclosure. *Fertility and Sterility, 82*, 172–179. doi:10.1016/j.fertnstert.2003.11.039

Lyerly, A. D., Steinhauser, K., Namey, E., Tulsky, J. A., Cook-Deegan, R., Sugarman, J., . . . Wallach, E. (2006). Factors that affect infertility patients' decisions about disposition of frozen embryos. *Fertility and Sterility, 85*, 1623–1630. doi:10.1016/j.fertnstert.2005.11.056

MacCallum, F., Golombok, S., & Brinsden, P. (2007). Parenting and child development in families with a child conceived through embryo donation. *Journal of Family Psychology, 21*, 278–287. doi:10.1037/0893-3200.21.2.278

MacDougall, K., Becker, G., Scheib, J. E., & Nachtigall, R. D. (2007). Strategies for disclosure: How parents approach telling their children that they were conceived with donor gametes. *Fertility and Sterility, 87*, 524–533. doi:10.1016/j.fertnstert.2006.07.1514

Mahalik, J. R., VanOrmer, E. A., & Simi, N. L. (2000). Ethical issues in using self-disclosure in feminist therapy. In M. M. Brabeck (Ed.), *Practicing feminist ethics in psychology* (pp. 189–201). Washington, DC: American Psychological Association. doi:10.1037/10343-009

Mahler, M., Pine, F., & Bergman, A. (1975). *The psychological birth of the human infant*. New York, NY: Basic Books.

Mahlstedt, P. P. (1985). The psychological component of infertility. *Fertility and Sterility, 43*, 335–346.

Mahlstedt, P. P. (1994). Psychological issues of infertility and assisted reproductive technology. *The Urologic Clinics of North America, 21*, 557–566.

Malik, S. H., & Coulson, N. S. (2008a). Computer-mediated infertility support groups: An exploratory study of online experiences. *Patient Education and Counseling, 73*, 105–113. doi:10.1016/j.pec.2008.05.024

Malik, S. H., & Coulson, N. S. (2008b). The male experience of infertility: A thematic analysis of an online infertility support group bulletin board. *Journal of Reproductive and Infant Psychology, 26,* 18–30. doi:10.1080/02646830701759777

Malin, M. (2003). Good, bad and troublesome: Infertility physicians' perceptions of women patients. *European Journal of Women's Studies, 10,* 301–319. doi:10.1177/1350506803010003004

Mannis, V. S. (1999). Single mothers by choice. *Family Relations, 48,* 121–128. doi:10.2307/585075

Markus, H., & Nurius, P. (1986). Possible selves. *American Psychologist, 41,* 954–969. doi:10.1037/0003-066X.41.9.954

Maroda, K. J. (2009). Less is more: An argument for the judicious use of self-disclosure. In A. Bloomgarden & R. B. Mennuti (Eds.), *Psychotherapist revealed* (pp. 17–29). New York, NY: Routledge.

Martin, T. L., & Doka, K. J. (2000). *Men don't cry . . . women do: Transcending gender stereotypes of grief.* Philadelphia, PA: Brunner/Mazel.

Matthews, T. J., & Ventura, S. J. (1997). Birth and fertility rates by educational attainment: United States, 1994. *Monthly Vital Statistics Report, 45*(Suppl.), 10.

Mayo Clinic. (1998–2009). *Varicocele.* Retrieved from http://www.mayoclinic.com/health/Varicocele/DS00618.

Mazor, A. (2004). Single motherhood via donor-insemination (DI): Separation, absence, and family creation. *Contemporary Family Therapy, 26,* 199–215. doi:10.1023/B:COFT.0000031243.42875.f4

Mazor, M. (1984). Emotional reactions to infertility. In M. Mazor & H. Simon (Eds.), *Infertility: Medical, emotional, and social considerations* (pp. 23–35). New York, NY: Human Science Press.

McAdams, D. P. (1993). *The stories we live by.* New York, NY: Guilford Press.

McGreal, D., Evans, B. J., & Burrows, G. D. (1997). Gender differences in coping following loss of a child through miscarriage or stillbirth: A pilot study. *Stress Medicine, 13,* 159–165. doi:10.1002/(SICI)1099-1700(199707)13:3<159::AID-SMI734>3.0.CO;2-5

McKinney, M., & Leary, K. (1999). Integrating quantitative and qualitative methods to study multifetal pregnancy reduction. *Journal of Women's Health, 8,* 259–268. doi:10.1089/jwh.1999.8.259

McLanahan, S., & Sandefur, G. (1994). *Growing up with a single parent: What hurts, what helps.* Cambridge, MA: Harvard University Press.

McMahon, C. A., Gibson, F. L., Leslie, G. I., Saunders, D. M., Porter, K. A., & Tennant, C. C. (2003). Embryo donation for medical research: Attitudes and concerns of potential donors. *Human Reproduction, 18,* 871–877. doi:10.1093/humrep/deg167

McManus, A. J., Hunter, L. P., & Renn, H. (2006). Lesbian experiences and needs during childbirth: Guidance for health care providers. *JOGNN, 35,* 13–23. doi:10.1111/J.1552-6909.2006.00008.x

McNaughton-Cassill, M. E., Bostwick, J. M., Arthur, N. J., Robinson, R. D., & Neal, G. S. (2002). Efficacy of brief couples support groups developed to manage the stress of in vitro fertilization treatment. *Mayo Clinic Proceedings, 77,* 1060–1066. doi:10.4065/77.10.1060

McQueeney, D. A., Stanton, A. L., & Sigmon, S. (1997). Efficacy of emotion-focused and problem-focused group therapies for women with fertility problems. *Journal of Behavioral Medicine, 20,* 313–331. doi:10.1023/A:1025560912766

McQuillan, J., Greil, A. L., White, L., & Jacob, M. C. (2003). Frustrated fertility: Infertility and psychological distress among women. *Journal of Marriage and the Family, 65,* 1007–1018. doi:10.1111/j.1741-3737.2003.01007.x

Medical Research Council Vitamin Study Research Group. (1991). Prevention of neural tube defects: Results of the Medical Research Council Vitamin Study. *The Lancet, 338,* 131–137.

Menning, B. E. (1976). RESOLVE: A support group for infertile couples. *The American Journal of Nursing, 76,* 258–259. doi:10.2307/3423816

Menning, B. E. (1980). The emotional needs of infertile couples. *Fertility and Sterility, 34,* 313–319.

Merari, D., Chetrit, A., & Modan, B. (2002). Emotional reactions and attitudes prior to in vitro fertilization: An inter-spouse study. *Psychology & Health, 17,* 629–640. doi:10.1080/08870440290025821

Middleton, W., Raphael, B., Martinek, N., & Misso, V. (1993). Pathological grief reactions. In: M. S. Stroebe, W. Stroebe, & R. O. Hansson (Eds.), *Handbook of bereavement* (pp. 44–61). Cambridge, England: Cambridge University Press.

Miller, J. B. (1966). *Toward a new psychology of women.* Boston, MA: Beacon Press.

Mooney-Somers, J., & Golombok, S. (2000). Children of lesbian mothers: From the 1970s to the new Millennium. *Sexual and Relationship Therapy, 15,* 121–126. doi:10.1080/14681990050010718

Morris, S. N., Missmer, S. A., Cramer, D. W., Powers, R. D., McShane, P. M., & Hornstein, M. D. (2006). Effects of lifetime exercise on the outcome of in vitro fertilization. *Obstetrics and Gynecology, 108,* 938–945.

Morse, C., & Van Hall, E. (1987). Psychosocial aspects of infertility: A review of current concepts. *Journal of Psychosomatic Obstetrics and Gynaecology, 6,* 157–164. doi:10.3109/01674828709019419

Murray, C., & Golombok, S. (2005a). Going it alone: Solo mothers and their infants conceived by donor insemination. *American Journal of Orthopsychiatry, 75,* 242–253. doi:10.1037/0002-9432.75.2.242

Murray, C., & Golombok, S. (2005b). Solo mothers and their donor insemination infants: Follow-up at age 2 years. *Human Reproduction, 20,* 1655–1660. doi:10.1093/humrep/deh823

Myers, D., & Hayes, J. A. (2006). Effects of therapist general self-disclosure and countertransference disclosure on ratings of the therapist and session. *Psychotherapy, 43,* 173–185. doi:10.1037/0033-3204.43.2.173

Nachtigall, R. D., Becker, G., Friese, C., Butler, A., & MacDougall, K. (2005). Parents' conceptualization of their frozen embryos complicates the disposition decision. *Fertility and Sterility, 84,* 431–434. doi:10.1016/j.fertnstert.2005.01.134

National Association of Social Workers. (1999). *NASW code of ethics.* Washington, DC: Author.

Navarro, M. (2008, September 7). The bachelor life includes a family. *The New York Times.* Retrieved from http://www.nytimes.com/2008/09/07/fashion/07single.html

Newman, B. M., & Newman, P. R. (1987). *Development through life.* Chicago, IL: Dorsey Press.

Newton, C. R., Fisher, J., Feyles, V., Tekpetey, F., Hughes, L., & Isacsson, D. (2007). Changes in patient preferences in the disposal of cryopreserved embryos. *Human Reproduction, 22,* 3124–3128. doi:10.1093/humrep/dem287

Newton, C. R., Sherrard, W., & Glavac, I. (1999). The fertility problem inventory: Measuring perceived infertility-related stress. *Fertility and Sterility, 72,* 54–62. doi:10.1016/S0015-0282(99)00164-8

Ogden, T. H. (1994). The analytic third: Working with intersubjective clinical facts. *The International Journal of Psycho-Analysis, 75,* 3–19.

O'Hara, M. H. (1997). The nature of postpartum depressive disorders. In L. Murray & P. J. Cooper (Eds.), *Postpartum depression and child development* (pp. 3–31). New York, NY: Guilford Press.

Oktay, K., Cil, A. P., & Bang, H. (2006). Efficiency of oocyte cryopreservation: A meta-analysis. *Fertility and Sterility, 86,* 70–80. doi:10.1016/j.fertnstert.2006.03.017

O'Leary, J., & Thorwick, C. (2006). Fathers' perspectives during pregnancy, post-perinatal loss. *JOGNN, 35,* 78–86.

Olshansky, E. F. (1990). Psychosocial implications of pregnancy after infertility. *NAACOG's Clinical Issues in Perinatal and Women's Health Nursing, 1,* 342–347.

Olshansky, E. (2003). A theoretical explanation for previously infertile mothers' vulnerability to depression. *Journal of Nursing Scholarship, 35,* 263–268. doi:10.1111/j.1547-5069.2003.00263.x

Olshansky, E., & Sereika, S. (2005). The transition from pregnancy to postpartum in previously infertile women: A focus on depression. *Archives of Psychiatric Nursing, 19,* 273–280. doi:10.1016/j.apnu.2005.08.003

Orenstein, P. (1995, June 18). Looking for a donor to call dad. *The New York Times Magazine.* Retrieved from http://www.peggyorenstein.com/articles/1995_donor_dad.html.

Orenstein, P. (2007, July 15). Your gamete, myself. *The New York Times Magazine.* Retrieved from http://www.nytimes.com/2007/07/15/magazine/15egg-t.html?pagewanted=1

Palomba, S., Giallauria, F., Falbo, A., Russo, T., Oppedisano, R., Tolino, A., . . . Orio, F. (2008). Structured exercise training programme versus hypocaloric hyperproteic diet in obese polycycstic ovary syndrome patients with anovulatory infertility: A 24-week pilot study. *Human Reproduction, 23,* 642–650.doi:10.1093/humrep/dem391

Parens, H. (1975). Parenthood as a developmental phase. *Journal of the American Psychoanalytic Association, 23,* 154–165.

Parks, C. A. (1998). Lesbian parenthood: A review of the literature. *American Orthopsychiatric Association, 68,* 376–389.

Patterson, C. J. (1992). Children of lesbian and gay parents. *Child Development, 63,* 1025–1042.

Patterson, C. J., & Redding, R. E. (1996). Lesbian and gay families with children: Implication of social science research for policy. *Journal of Social Issues, 52,* 29–50.

Paulus, W. E., Zhang, M., Strehler, E., El-Danasouri, I., & Sterzik, K. (2002). Influence of acupuncture on the pregnancy rate in patients who undergo assisted reproduction therapy. *Fertility and Sterility, 77,* 721–724. doi:10.1016/S0015-0282(01)03273-3

Pei, J., Strehler, E., Noss, U., Abt, M., Piomboni, P., Baccetti, B., & Sterzik, K. (2005). Quantitative evaluation of spermatozoa ultrastructure after acupuncture treatment for idiopathic male infertility. *Fertility and Sterility, 84,* 141–147. doi:10.1016/j.fertnstert.2004.12.056

Pepe, M. V., & Byrne, T. J. (1991). Women's perceptions of immediate and long-term effects of failed infertility treatment on marital and sexual satisfaction. *Family Relations, 40,* 303–309. doi:10.2307/585016

Peppers, L. G., & Knapp, R. J. (1980). *Motherhood and mourning: Perinatal death.* New York, NY: Praeger Publishers.

Peterson, B. D., Newton, C. R., & Feingold, T. (2007). Anxiety and sexual stress in men and women undergoing infertility treatment. *Fertility and Sterility, 88,* 911–914. doi:10.1016/j.fertnstert.2006.12.023

Peterson, Z. D. (2002). More than a mirror: The ethics of therapist self-disclosure. *Psychotherapy, 39,* 21–31. doi:10.1037/0033-3204.39.1.21

Pines, D. (1972). Pregnancy and motherhood: Interaction between fantasy and reality. *The British Journal of Medical Psychology, 45,* 333–343.

Pines, D. (1990). Pregnancy, miscarriage, and abortion: A psychoanalytic perspective. *The International Journal of Psycho-Analysis, 71,* 301–307.

Puddifoot, J. E., & Johnson, M. P. (1999). Active grief, despair and difficulty coping: Some measured characteristics of male response following their partner's miscarriage. *Journal of Reproductive and Infant Psychology, 17,* 89–93. doi:10.1080/02646839908404587

Ralt, D. (1999). Qi, information and the net of life. *Acupuncture in Medicine, 17,* 131–133. doi:10.1136/aim.17.2.131

Rando, T. A. (1985). Bereaved parents: Particular difficulties, unique factors, and treatment issues. *Social Work, 30,* 19–23.

Rando, T. (1986). *Parental loss of a child.* Champaign, IL: Research Press.

Reardon, D. C., & Cougle, J. R. (2002). Depression and unintended pregnancy in the National Longitudinal Survey of Youth: A cohort study. *British Medical Journal, 324*, 151–152. doi:10.1136/bmj.324.7330.151

Reardon, D. C., Cougle, J. R., Rue, V. M., Shuping, M. W., Coleman, P. K., & Ney, P. G. (2003). Psychiatric admissions of low-income women following abortion and childbirth. *Canadian Medical Association Journal, 168*, 1253–1256.

Reid, M. (2007). The loss of a baby and the birth of the next infant: The mother's experience. *Journal of Child Psychotherapy, 33*, 181–201. doi:10.1080/00754170701431339

Resch, M., Szendei, G., & Haasz, P. (2004). Bulimia from a gynecological view: Hormonal changes. *Journal of Obstetrics & Gynaecology, 24*, 907–910. doi:10.1080/01443610400018924

RESOLVE, The National Infertility Organization. (2008a). *Frequently asked questions about infertility.* Retrieved from http://www.resolve.org/site/PageServer?pagename=lrn_wii_faq

RESOLVE, The National Infertility Organization. (2008b). *Secondary infertility.* Retrieved from http://www.resolve.org/site/PageServer?pagename=lrn_wii_si

Roberts, P., & Newton, P. M. (1987). Levinsonian studies of women's adult development. *Psychology and Aging, 2*, 154–163. doi:10.1037/0882-7974.2.2.154

Robertson, E., Grace, S., Wallington, T., & Stewart, D. E. (2004). Antenatal risk factors for postpartum depression: A synthesis of recent literature. *General Hospital Psychiatry, 26*, 289–295. doi:10.1016/j.genhosppsych.2004.02.006

Robertson, J. A. (2003). Extending preimplantation genetic diagnosis: Medical and non-medical uses. *Journal of Medical Ethics, 29*, 213–216. doi:10.1136/jme.29.4.213

Robinson, M., Baker, L., & Nackerud, L. (1999). The relationship of attachment theory and perinatal loss. *Death Studies, 23*, 257–270. doi:10.1080/074811899201073

Rogers, C. (1951). *On becoming a person.* Boston, MA: Houghton Mifflin.

Rothaupt, J., & Becker, K. (2007). A literature review of Western bereavement theory: From decathecting to continuing bonds. *The Family Journal, 15*, 6–15. doi:10.1177/1066480706294031

Rubin, H. (2002). The impact and meaning of childlessness: An interview study of childless women. *Dissertation Abstracts International: Section B. Sciences and Engineering, 62*(8-B).

Rubin, R. (1975). Maternal tasks in pregnancy. *Maternal-Child Nursing Journal, 4*, 143–153.

Sachs, P. L., & Burns, L. H. (2006). Recipient counseling for oocyte donation. In S. N. Covington & L. H. Burns (Eds.), *Infertility counseling: A comprehensive handbook for clinicians* (2nd ed., pp. 319–338). New York, NY: Cambridge University Press.

Salter-Ling, N., Hunter, M., & Glover, L. (2001). Donor insemination: Exploring the experience of treatment and intention to tell. *Journal of Reproductive and Infant Psychology, 19*, 175–186. doi:10.1080/02646830120073198

Salzer, L. P. (2000). Adoption after infertility. In L. H. Burns & S. N. Covington (Eds.), *Infertility counseling: A comprehensive handbook for clinicians*. New York, NY: The Parthenon Publishing Group.

Sandelowski, M., Harris, B. G., & Black, B. P. (1992). Relinquishing infertility: The work of pregnancy for infertile couples. *Qualitative Health Research, 2*, 282–301. doi:10.1177/104973239200200303

Sandelowski, M., Harris, B. G., & Holditch-Davis, D. (1993). "Somewhere out there:" Parental claiming in the preadoption waiting period. *Journal of Contemporary Ethnography, 21*, 464–486. doi:10.1177/089124193021004003

Sandelowski, M., & Pollock, C. (1986). Women's experiences of infertility. *Journal of Nursing Scholarship, 18*, 140–144. doi:10.1111/j.1547-5069.1986.tb00563.x

Santona, A., & Zavattini, G. C. (2005). Partnering and parenting expectations in adoptive couples. *Sexual and Relationship Therapy, 20*, 309–322. doi:10.1080/14681990500142004

Schectman, K. W. (1980). Motherhood as an adult developmental stage. *American Journal of Psychoanalysis, 40*, 273–281.

Schectman, M. (1996). *The constitution of selves*. Ithaca, NY: Cornell University.

Scher, A., Petterson, B., Blair, E., Ellenberg, J., Grether, J. K., Haan, E., . . . Nelson, K. (2002). The risk of mortality or cerebral palsy in twins: A collaborative population-based study. *Pediatric Research, 52*, 671–681.

Schut, H. A. W., Stroebe, M., de Keijser, J., & van den Bout, J. (1997). Intervention for the bereaved: Gender differences in the efficacy of grief counseling. *The British Journal of Clinical Psychology, 36*, 63–72.

Serrano, F., & Lima, M. L. (2006). Recurrent miscarriage: Psychological and relational consequences for couples. *Psychology and Psychotherapy, 79*, 585–594.

Shanley, M. L. (2002). Collaboration and commodification in assisted procreation: Reflections on an open market and anonymous donation in human sperm and eggs (Special issue). *Law & Society Review. 36*, 257–284.

Shapiro, C. H. (1988). *Infertility and pregnancy loss: A guide for helping professionals*. San Francisco, CA: Jossey-Bass.

Sherman, S., Eltes, F., Wolfson, V., Zabludovsky, N., & Bartoov, B. (1997). Effect of acupuncture on sperm parameters of males suffering from subfertility related to low sperm quality. *Archives of Andrology, 39*, 155–161. doi:10.3109/01485019708987914

Simon, B., Lee, S. J., Partridge, A. H., & Runowicz, C. D. (2005). Preserving fertility after cancer. *CA: A Cancer Journal for Clinicians, 55*, 211–228. doi:10.3322/canjclin.55.4.211

Single Mothers by Choice. (2007). *Single mothers by choice*. Retrieved from http://www.singlemothersbychoice.com/

Slade, P., Emery, J., & Lieberman, B. A. (1997). A prospective, longitudinal study of emotions and relationships in in-vitro fertilization treatment. *Human Reproduction, 12*, 183–190. doi:10.1093/humrep/12.1.183

Smith, C., Coyle, M., & Norman, R. J. (2006). Influence of acupuncture stimulation on pregnancy rates for women undergoing embryo transfer. *Fertility and Sterility*, *85*, 1352–1358. doi:10.1016/j.fertnstert.2005.12.015

Sophie, J. (1987). Internalized homophobia and lesbian identity. *Journal of Homosexuality*, *14*, 53–65. doi:10.1300/J082v14n01_05

Spallanzani, L. (1784). *Dissertations relative to the natural history of animals and vegetables* (T. Beddons, Trans.,Vol. 2, pp. 195–199). London, England: J. Murray.

Spiegel, D., Bloom, J. R., Kraemer, H. C., & Gottheil, E. (1989). Effect of psychosocial treatment on survival of patients with metastatic breast cancer. *The Lancet*, *334*, 888–891. doi:10.1016/S0140-6736(89)91551-1

Stewart, W. (1977). *A psychosocial study of the formation of the early adult life structure in women* (Unpublished doctoral dissertation). Columbia University, New York, NY.

Stinson, K. M., Lasker, J. N., Lohmann, J., & Toedter, L. J. (1992). Parents' grief following pregnancy loss: A comparison of mothers and fathers. *Family Relations*, *41*, 218–223. doi:10.2307/584836

Storey, A. E., Walsh, C. J., Quinton, R. L., & Wynne-Edwards, K. E. (2000). Hormonal correlates of paternal responsiveness in new and expectant fathers. *Evolution and Human Behavior*, *21*, 79–95. doi:10.1016/S1090-5138(99)00042-2

Strauss, R., & Goldberg, W. A. (1999). Self and possible selves during the transition to fatherhood. *Journal of Family Psychology*, *13*, 244–259. doi:10.1037/0893-3200.13.2.244

Stricker, G. (2003). The many faces of self-disclosure. *Journal of Clinical Psychology*, *59*, 623–630.

Stroebe, M., & Schut, H. (1999). The dual process model of coping with bereavement: Rationale and description. *Death Studies*, *23*, 197–224. doi:10.1080/074811899201046

Swanson, P. B., Pearsall-Jones, J. G., & Hay, D. A. (2002). How mothers cope with the death of a twin or higher multiple. *Twin Research*, *5*, 156–164. doi:10.1375/136905202320227808

Tasker, F., & Golombok, S. (1997). *Growing up in a lesbian family*. New York, NY: Guilford.

The International Council on Infertility Information Dissemination. (1992–2008). Infertility basics. Retrieved from www.inciid.org/printpage.php?cat=infertility 101&id=262

Thorn, P. (2006). Recipient counseling for donor insemination. In S. N. Covington & L. H. Burns (Eds.), *Infertility counseling: A comprehensive handbook for clinicians* (2nd ed., pp. 305–318). New York, NY: Cambridge University Press.

Toedter, L. J., Lasker, J. N., & Alhadeff, M. A. (1988). The Perinatal Grief Scale: Development and initial validation. *American Journal of Orthopsychiatry*, *58*, 435–449.

Turton, P., Badenhorst, W., Hughes, P., Ward, J., Riches, S., & White, S. (2006). Psychological impact of stillbirth on fathers in the subsequent pregnancy and puerperium. *The British Journal of Psychiatry, 188,* 165–172. doi:10.1192/bjp.188.2.165

Valentine, D. P. (1986). Psychological impact of infertility: Identifying issues and needs. *Social Work in Health Care, 11,* 61–69. doi:10.1300/J010v11n04_05

Van Berkel, D., Candido, A., & Pijffers, W. H. (2007). Becoming a mother by non-anonymous egg donation: Secrecy and the relationship between egg recipient, egg donor and egg donation child. *Journal of Psychosomatic Obstetrics and Gynae-cology, 28,* 97–104. doi:10.1080/01674820701409868

Van Putten, R., & LaWall, J. (1981). Postpartum psychosis in an adoptive mother and in a father. *Psychosomatics, 22,* 1087–1089.

Verhaak, C. M., Smeenk, J. M. J., van Minnen, A., Kremer, J. A. M., & Kraaimaat, F. W. (2005). A longitudinal, prospective study on emotional adjustment before, during and after consecutive fertility treatment cycles. *Human Reproduction, 20,* 2253–2260. doi:10.1093/humrep/dei015

Vieira, T. (2002). When joy becomes grief: Screening tools for postpartum depression. *AWHONN Lifelines, 6,* 506–513. doi:10.1177/1091592302239621

Wang, W., Check, J. H., Liss, J., & Choe, J. K. (2005). A matched controlled study to evaluate the efficacy of acupuncture for improving pregnancy rates following in vitro fertilization-embryo transfer. *Fertility and Sterility, 83,* S24. doi:10.1016/j.fertnstert.2005.01.021

Warner, J. (2008, January 3). Outsourced wombs. *The New York Times.* Retrieved from http://opinionator.blogs.nytimes.com/2008/01/03/outsourced-wombs/

Watson, R. I. (2005). When the patient has experienced severe trauma. In A. Rosen & J. Rosen (Eds.), *Frozen dreams: Psychodynamic dimensions of infertility and assisted reproduction* (pp. 219–235). Hillsdale, NJ: Analytic Press.

Watt, H. (2004). Preimplantation genetic diagnosis: Choosing the "good enough" child. *Health Care Analysis, 12,* 51–60. doi:10.1023/B:HCAN.0000026653.01543.3a

Weinraub, M., Horvath, D. L., & Gringlas, M. B. (2002). Single parenthood. In M. H. Bornstein (Ed.), *Handbook of parenting: Being and becoming a parent* (Vol. 3, 2nd ed., pp. 109–140). Hillsdale, NJ: Erlbaum.

Westergaard, L. G., Mao, Q., Krogslund, M., Sandrini, S., Lenz, S., & Grinsted, J. (2006). Acupuncture on the day of embryo transfer significantly improves the reproductive outcome in infertile women: A prospective randomized trial. *Fertility and Sterility, 85,* 1341–1346. doi:10.1016/j.fertnstert.2005.08.070

Williams, L., Bischoff, R., & Ludes, J. (1992). A biopsychosocial model for treating infertility. *Contemporary Family Therapy, 14,* 309–322. doi:10.1007/BF00891868

Williams, R. L., & Medalie, J. H. (1994). Twins: Double pleasure or double trouble? *American Family Physician, 49,* 869–876.

Wilson, A. L., Fenton, L. J., Stevens, D. C., & Soule, D. J. (1982). The death of a newborn twin: An analysis of parental bereavement. *Pediatrics, 70,* 587–591.

Wingert, S., Harvey, C. D. H., Duncan, K. A., & Berry, R. E. (2005). Assessing the needs of assisted reproductive technology users of an online bulletin board. *Inter-*

national Journal of Consumer Studies, 29, 468–478. doi:10.1111/j.1470-6431. 2005.00461.x

Wisner, K. L., Chambers, C., & Sit, D. K. Y. (2006). Postpartum depression: A major public health problem. *Journal of the American Medical Association, 296,* 2616–2618. doi:10.1001/jama.296.21.2616

Withrow, R., & Schwiebert, V. L. (2005). Twin loss: Implications for counselors working with surviving twins. *Journal of Counseling and Development, 83,* 21–28.

Wright, J., Duchesne, C., Sabourin, S., Bissonnette, F., Benoit, J., & Girard, Y. (1991). Psychosocial distress and infertility: Men and women respond differently. *Fertility and Sterility, 55,* 100–108.

Wurn, B. F., Wurn, L. J., King, C. R., Heuer, M. A., Roscow, A. S., Hornberger, K., & Scharf, E. S. (2008). Treating fallopian tube occlusion with a manual pelvic physical therapy. *Alternative Therapies in Health and Medicine, 14,* 18–23.

Wynne-Edwards, K. E. (2001). Hormonal changes in mammalian fathers. *Hormones and Behavior, 40,* 139–145. doi:10.1006/hbeh.2001.1699

Zeanah, C. H., Dailey, J. V., Rosenblatt, M., & Saller, D. N. (1993). Do women grieve after terminating pregnancies because of fetal anomalies? A controlled investigation. *Obstetrics and Gynecology, 82,* 270–275.

Zhang, M., Huang, G., Lu, F., Paulus, W. E., & Sterzik, K. (2002). Influence of acupuncture on idiopathic male infertility in assisted reproductive technology. *Journal of Huazhong University of Science and Technology Medical Sciences, 22,* 228–230.

Zheng, Z. (1997). Analysis on the therapeutic effect of combined use of acupuncture and medication in 297 cases of male sterility. *Journal of Traditional Chinese Medicine, 17,* 190–193.

Zicklin, G. (1995). Deconstructing legal rationality: The case of lesbian and gay family relationships. *Marriage & Family Review, 21,* 55–76. doi:10.1300/J002v21n03_04

Zlotogora, J. (2002). Parental decisions to abort or continue a pregnancy with an abnormal finding after an invasive prenatal test. *Prenatal Diagnosis, 22,* 1102–1106. doi:10.1002/pd.472

Zur, O. (2009). Therapist self-disclosure: Standard of care, ethical considerations, and therapeutic context. In A. Bloomgarden & R. B. Menutti (Eds.), *Psychotherapist revealed* (pp. 31–51). New York, NY: Routledge.

Zweifel, J., Christianson, M., Jaeger, A. S., Olive, D., & Lindheim, S. R. (2007). Needs assessment for those donating to stem cell research. *Fertility and Sterility, 88,* 560–564. doi:10.1016/j.fertnstert.2006.12.042

INDEX

ABOUT THE AUTHORS

Janet Jaffe, PhD, a clinical psychologist in San Diego, California, is cofounder and codirector of the Center for Reproductive Psychology. She has served as an adjunct faculty member at the California School of Professional Psychology at Alliant International University, is a member of the American Society for Reproductive Medicine, and has presented at conferences across the country on the psychology of the reproductive process, both to professional organizations and to the general public. Dr. Jaffe is coauthor of *Unsung Lullabies, Understanding and Coping With Infertility* (2005). Currently in private practice, Dr. Jaffe specializes in the issues of loss and bereavement related to miscarriage, infertility, and other reproductive trauma.

Martha O. Diamond, PhD, received her bachelor's degree in psychology from Stanford University and her doctorate in clinical psychology from the University of Michigan. She is cofounder and codirector of the Center for Reproductive Psychology in San Diego, California. Dr. Diamond is coauthor of *Unsung Lullabies, Understanding and Coping With Infertility* (2005). In addition to her clinical practice, Dr. Diamond has lectured nationally and internationally on reproductive issues, including the psychological trauma of infertility, miscarriage, and premature or complicated births. She also conducts in-service training for medical professionals on the psychological impact of adverse reproductive events and the emotional needs of their reproductive patients.